SIMPLY FOR THE LOVE OF IT:

A BEGINNER'S GUIDE TO SUPPORT SERVICES FOR PEOPLE WITH DEVELOPMENTAL DISABILITIES

James B. McKelvey

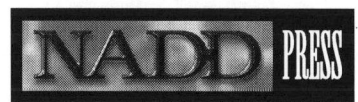

® Copyright 2003
NADD Press
132 Fair St.
Kingston, NY 12401

All rights reserved

No part of this book may be reproduced, stored in a retrieval system, or transmitted, in any form, or by any means, electronic, mechanical, photocopying, microfilming, recording, or otherwise, without written permission from the Publisher.

Printed in the United States of America

Trademarks: A number of product and brand names for which the author and publisher have reason to believe trademark, service marks, or other proprietary rights may exist have been designated as such by use of initial capitalization. However, no attempt has been made to designate as trademarks or service marks all words or terms which are commonly used as a reference to a generic concept or practice in which proprietary rights might exist. The inclusion or exclusion or definition of a word or term is not intended to affect, or to express any judgment on, the validity or legal status of any proprietary right which may be claimed in that word or term.

Gender references are intentionally varied and represent no significant implication.

Library of Congress Cataloging in Publication Data
McKelvey, James B.
Simply for the Love of It: A Beginners Guide to Support Services for People with Developmental Disabilities / James B. McKelvey

p. cm
Includes appendices
ISBN 1-57256-037-1
1. Developmental Disabilities. 2. Community services for people with disabilities.
3. History of services to people with disabilities. 4. Staff training resources.

CONTENTS

Chapter 1
BEGINNER'S MIND 1

Chapter 2
LEARNING FROM THE PAST 8

Chapter 3
FROM INSTITUTION TO INCLUSION 21

Chapter 4
LIFE PLANNING—THEN AND NOW 37

Chapter 5
"MENTAL RETARDATION" RECONSIDERED 56

Chapter 6
THE ABC'S OF LEARNING 73

Chapter 7
TEACHING REAL SKILLS FOR THE REAL WORLD 87

Chapter 8
MENTAL ILLNESS AND ITS TREATMENTS 104

Chapter 9
"WHY DOES SHE ACT THAT WAY?"—
UNDERSTANDING CHALLENGING BEHAVIOR 126

Chapter 10
A MATTER OF RIGHTS 152

Chapter 11
SEX, SMOKES AND THE RESPONSIBLE ADULT 169

Chapter 12
DISABILITIES THROUGH THE LIFECYCLE 189

Chapter 13
A HOME AND A JOB IN THE REAL WORLD 210

Chapter 14
WHAT'S LOVE GOT TO DO WITH IT? 230

Appendix I
GLOSSARY OF TERMS 239

Appendix II
RESOURCES (WHERE TO GO FOR MORE INFORMATION) 257

Chapter 1

BEGINNER'S MIND

I didn't get into this business on purpose.

It all started in the spring of 1977. I had survived my first winter as a back-to-the-land country hippie in an old farmhouse on a ridge in northern West Virginia. I had moved to the country to try to "get myself together." To a kid raised in the suburbs of Chicago, that first winter had brought painful lessons in heating with wood, driving in mud, and living without electricity or running water. As the last snow melted my road into an ooze of mud, I decided I needed a job.

There aren't many jobs in rural West Virginia that require the skills of a person with a bachelor's degree in Philosophy, a Master's of Divinity from Harvard, and four years experience as a Unitarian-Universalist minister. Coal mining and timbering were rough jobs that you couldn't get into unless your Daddy had worked there. But there was a place an hour south of where I lived that seemed to hold some promise of employment.

The place was called Colin Anderson Center, a campus-like scattering of buildings on the banks of the Ohio River just north of the small town of St. Marys. All I knew about it, from the reports of friends, was that it was a state-run facility for what they called "retarded kids." I wasn't sure what that meant. As far as I could remember, the only "retarded kid" I had ever known was the girl in our neighborhood who used to repeat whatever us kids yelled at her. Sometimes she stood out in the street repeating her name. We thought it was funny. Our parents told us we should leave her alone because she was "retarded."

I stopped by the Personnel Office at Colin Anderson Center one day and they signed me up to be a "direct care" staff person—a Psychiatric Aide I. I didn't know what direct care was. I had a lot to learn.

LEARNING "DIRECT CARE"

Even though I had a lot of education, I was totally inexperienced in "direct care." I was going to need some training. So on my first day of work, I reported to the "Basic Aide Training" class in the Staff Development building. For the next week my classmates and I learned how to make a bed with hospital corners, how to mop floors and change diapers, how to feed with a nasogastric tube, how to give enemas (both soap suds and Fleets).

You see, Colin Anderson Center was, at that time, run like a hospital. Doctors and nurses were in charge, and the main point of the place was to keep "the residents" safe and healthy...to take care of them. That's why we learned a lot about how to clean up vomit, drool, urine and feces and how to protect ourselves from infection. That's why we learned seizure management, "protective restraint" to keep people from hurting themselves, and CPR, in case they stopped breathing.

After "taking care," the second most important job of a Psychiatric Aide was to keep people under control. A staff Psychologist taught us a class on "The ABC's of Behavior Modification." In that class, I learned we would be running training programs written by the psychologists, using rewards and punishments to shape new behavior. It was all based on some psychological theory called Behaviorism.

I finished my week of training and a few days of orientation, where I had to spend one day in different parts of the Center—the Big Boys Ward, Boys Cottage, and the Crib Building. My final assignment was 127 North Crib, a ward that housed 35 non-ambulatory adults. "Nonambulatory" meant they didn't walk, so everyone who lived on that ward spent most of their time in wheelchairs. I worked second shift (2:30-11:00 PM) with one other staff person.

I learned something new every day of my work at Colin Anderson Center, but many of the ways we did things left me confused. Some of my confusion was due to the fact that I didn't know the history of how a place like Colin Anderson Center got to be the way it was. I didn't know that, bad as conditions seemed at the time, there had been times when things had been much worse. I didn't know people were working around the world to raise awareness of the rights of people living in institutions. I didn't know the reasons for the training programs and the separation of the wards. And I didn't understand why the people I worked with, people who were said to have mental retardation, acted the way they did. I was working in one facility, with its own culture and rules and problems. I didn't know what had happened in the past or what was possible in the future.

If you're new to the field of providing supports to people who have developmental disabilities, you may also wonder how all of this work we do came about. Even if you've been working in the field for a number of years, you may have been tossed into the middle of things without having the opportunity to get an overview of the history and the issues of supports for people who have developmental disabilities. That's where this book comes in.

A theme throughout this book will be—where we've been, where we are, and where we could go. Developing the best supports for people with developmental disabilities is an ongoing process. Over the years, many people have dedicated their lives to finding better ways of doing things. Twenty years later those "better ways" may look backward and quaint. You are now part of the process. But you needn't reinvent the wheel. I'll tell you about some of the territory that's been covered, celebrate the good things that are happening now, and point you in the direction of needed improvements.

TEACHERS AND FRIENDS

Over the years I worked at Colin Anderson Center, I learned a lot from psychologists, social workers and special education teachers who had studied their field in college. I borrowed books from them, asked them questions, and gradually filled in some of the gaps in my knowledge.

But I learned most from the people who lived at Colin Anderson Center. I got to know many of them as friends and was always amazed at their ability to use their personal resources to put together some kind of life for themselves. They were the people who made my work interesting and rewarding.

Some of the people I remember most fondly include Raymond, whose clever pranks with the new fire alarm boxes drove a newly graduated psychologist back to graduate school.

And Olive, who had the reputation as the terror of Girls' Cottage when I first met her. Over the years, she transferred to a new program where she learned the rewards of getting along with people...and became a person other people liked.

And Bonnie, who everyday asked me where the moon was and complained that she didn't get any "mail call."

And Billy, who, because of his cerebral palsy, spent his life lying on a homemade plywood cart with bicycle wheels and who had a crush on every female staff person.

The woman who was to be my wife worked in the Recreation Department at Colin Anderson Center. She got interested in helping Billy dictate the story of his life. It was a slow and often frustrating process, because Billy's speech was so hard to understand. But the story grew day by day, a heartbreaking story of abandonment and abuse.

One year we had Billy out to our newly renovated schoolhouse for Christmas. We helped him sip wine (which greatly improved the clarity of his speech), and we took him for a ride across the backcountry ridges, his new personal care chair strapped in the back of my pickup truck for the view of his life.

And Lloyd, my favorite, whose happy grin was surrounded by layers of scar tissue from thousands of seizures that caused him to fall suddenly, hitting his chin.

Lloyd came out to the house, too; and we both laughed hysterically as I taught him that out in the country it's OK for men to pee in the bushes.

These people became my friends and my teachers. I learned from them how difficult it is to overcome not only a disability but also the prejudice and isolation inflicted by the community at large, as well as by the so-called "experts".

And I learned what miracles can occur just through offering a person the opportunity to have a "real life in the real world."

That was almost 25 years ago. Colin Anderson Center has been shut down, and all the people who lived there have moved to community residences. I thank them for all they taught me, and I hope they're all having wonderful lives.

BEGINNER'S MINDS

When I started my work at Colin Anderson Center, my ignorance about everything made me insecure. I was used to being an "expert," someone who could speak knowledgeably about my work. Suddenly, I was a beginner.

But I learned that being a beginner isn't so bad. Zen Master Shunryu Suzuki once said, "In the beginner's mind there are many possibilities, but in the expert's there are few." If you are a beginner in the field of providing supports for people with disabilities, rejoice! Your mind is not already full of "expert" notions of how things should be done. Your mind is full of possibilities.

Don't be intimidated by professionals who think you don't know what you're doing unless you have a lot of college degrees. Support services is something you know more "by heart" than in your head. Sure, there's stuff to be learned; and this book is a good place to start. When you've read through the material and looked into any of the suggested resources that might interest you, you'll know more than you did when you started. But, regardless of how much you learn, never lose your "beginner's mind."

Because it is a "Beginner's Guide," the material in this book is, necessarily, oversimplified. Each chapter could be expanded into several books. If you want to explore any area in more depth, you can refer to the "Resources" listed in Appendix II at the end of the book.

Whether you are just starting to work in this field or have had years of experience, whether you are a family member of a person with disabilities or are learning how to live with your own disability, whether you do this professionally or as a volunteer, this book will serve to give you the lay of the land. I'll share some history, some stories, some tips and techniques that will assist you in your work.

Some of the topics dealt with in the book bring up issues that are controversial. Wherever that is the case, I will try to show you the history of the issue and what's at stake in the decisions involved. I will also sometimes admit that where I'm coming from is based on my own prejudice (yes; we all have them) and experience.

I have very consciously shied away from the voiceless tone of the usual textbook. In this book, you will know who is speaking. I care about this stuff, and I'm outspoken. I hope you will be too. I encourage you to form your own opinions on these matters, based on what you see for yourself. If you don't care about these things, you'll never amount to much as a support services provider. You can keep up with the latest information and opinions on these issues by visiting the websites listed in the "Resources" section.

A NOTE ABOUT NAMES AND TERMS

I use a lot of first names in the telling of stories throughout this book. Some of them are the actual names of the person the story is about. Others are made up. It doesn't matter which is which. The stories are all based on real experiences I've had doing this kind of work. You'll develop your own stories...with names of new friends attached.

The philosophy of what I call "Real Life in the Real World" for people with disabilities emphasizes the universal (applied equally to all) qualities of all people. This universal nature goes for language, as well. I think we should be careful to stay away from professional jargon that serves only to emphasize differences and often puts people in boxes of separation. It's important, though, that you understand some of the terms the professionals use. When new terms are introduced, they will be defined clearly. Other words that may be strange to you, can be found in the Glossary at the back of the book. If you forget what something means, you can always look back at the Glossary (it's not cheating).

SIMPLY FOR THE LOVE OF IT

One afternoon, driving home after a long day dealing with problems at several group homes, I was listening to Don Henley's 1984 CD "Building The Perfect Beast." Stuck in the middle of songs of Los Angeles desolation is the poignant "A Month of Sundays." That song about the loss of American farms and of small town life always chokes me up a little. That particular day, though, I was struck by one line: "Folks these days just don't do nothin' simply for the love of it."

There is a deeper value in doing something for the love of it, something that gives meaning to your life and is worth doing.

Doesn't that strike you as true? A lot of people seem to do what they do so they can be rich and famous or to beat the other guy. The song, though, is suggesting that there is a deeper value in doing something for the love of it, doing work that gives meaning to your life and improves the lives of others.

You have the opportunity to do that kind of work. You can make a difference in someone's life and be part of making this a better world for all of us to live in. You may get a paycheck for your work, or you may do it only because it means something deep to you. But you will always, in the end, do it because of the people involved..."simply for the love of it."

The real stuff has to come from you. In order to be successful, you've got to bring to this work a heart of compassion, an enormous amount of patience, and a great love of people. But, oh, what success it can be!

Chapter 2

LEARNING FROM THE PAST

The philosopher George Santayana wrote, "Those who cannot remember the past are condemned to repeat it." There are some things about the way we've related to people who have disabilities that certainly shouldn't be done again. But unless you know about where we've been, you won't really understand the exciting new places we're going.

There is a theme running throughout this book—what we did in the past, what we do now, and what we could be doing in the future. I've already shared with you a bit of my personal past. That personal history is important not because of who I am as the author of this book but because it is representative of the process of learning from our experience and improving our work day by day. If you're just starting out working with people who have disabilities, you can benefit from knowing the journey we've taken in our understanding of who they are and what they need. You are now part of that journey. You will take us into what I hope will be a glorious future.

This chapter is about the history of how people who have disabilities have been viewed and how they've been treated. It's not a complete history, by any means. It's just some of the highlights I've found interesting as I've tried to put my experience into the context of where we've been and where we might be going.

EARLY DAYS

Sometimes while I was working at Colin Anderson Center I would wonder about what life would be like for people like Raymond and Olive in the long past. Did primitive people take care of those among them who were different? Or did they just leave them behind or cast them out? We'll probably never know. As bad as some of the things about Colin Anderson Center were, at least the people who lived there were given shelter and food and medical care.

Throughout most of early history, people with mental disorders were thought of as possessed by spirits. If their behavior wasn't too harmful, they might be seen as blessed by guiding angels. If their actions were troublesome, though, the possession was seen as from the devil. Many people who were persecuted as witches probably had some sort of mental disorder.

One of the earliest attempts at caring for people who had what we now call developmental or mental disorders was St. Mary's of Bethlehem Hospital, opened in London, England in 1414. It was called an "asylum," the word meaning "sanctuary, refuge, and protection." It wasn't a hospital in the sense that we know it today. There were no doctors or treatments. Unfortunately for those who were placed in Bethlehem, there was no safety or protection either. People from town often visited the asylum to be entertained by the behavior of the inmates. Gambling, prostitution and various forms of abuse were common. The conditions were so bad that we got a new word from the shortened name of the hospital—Bedlam, which means "a scene of uproar and confusion."

CUTTING THE CHAINS

It wasn't until the late 18th century, the Age of Enlightenment, that some people started studying the causes of mental disorders with a view to try to help the people who were affected by them. In places like Bedlam in London and the Bicetre in Paris, the inmates were often chained and shackled. Their strange behavior was seen as dangerous. Phillipe Pinel (pin-EL), the leading psychiatrist of his day, was the first to see mental disorders as diseases rather than curses. In 1793 he took the chains off the people in the French asylums and began to treat them humanely and supportively. More than 200 years ago, Pinel realized treating people badly only made their condition worse. He must have been someone who did his work "for the love of it."

ITARD AND THE WILD BOY

Another pioneer working at the same time as Pinel was Jean Marc Itard (ee-TAR). Itard was a physician and teacher at the National Institute for the Deaf and Dumb in Paris. He and others had been developing new teaching methods for children who had hearing and vision impairments. Itard believed these children didn't just need care and protection. He believed they could learn.

In 1799, Itard found an 11-year-old boy roaming naked in the woods near Paris. The boy had apparently been abandoned by his parents. He had never learned to speak or understand French, and he acted like a wild animal. Itard named the boy Victor, but he was to become famous as 'The Wild Boy of Aveyron.'

Itard was fascinated with the boy and invented his own techniques to teach Victor social and communication skills. For example, Itard drew pictures of common objects—a shoe, a pencil, a book—and tacked them to the wall. He would then tell Victor, "Get the shoe" (in French, of course). Victor would find a shoe and hang it on the nail next to the picture. Later, Itard replaced the pictures with words, and Victor began to learn to read.

Itard's work is important because he saw people who had trouble learning not as failures or unfortunates but as a challenge to the abilities of the teacher. It's not that they can't learn; it's that we haven't learned how to teach them. Itard's teaching techniques are the forerunners of many of today's special education procedures.

SEGUIN'S "SCHOOL FOR IDIOTS"

Edward Seguin (suh-GAN) was another French teacher who studied Itard's new methods in Paris. He was particularly interested in children who were known as "idiots" or "feebleminded." These are the English terms, but the French is similar. They are words that are offensive to today's ears. Imagine calling someone an idiot or a moron today! In those days, though, the terms were considered scientific descriptions of particular characteristics. A "moron" (from the Greek word for "foolish") was someone with mental retardation in what we would now call the 'Mild' range. An "imbecile" (from the Latin meaning "without support") was someone in today's Moderate range. And an "idiot" (from the Latin meaning "ignorant person") was on the lowest level, what we now call "Severe and Profound." The use of these categories and the terms that described them was seen at the time as an advance in understanding. It was state of the art best practice.

It took a lot of work for Seguin to get the support needed to open his "School for Idiots" in Paris in 1842. Seguin believed mental disorders were the result of "weakness" of the brain and nerves and senses, so his educational program consisted largely of physical exercises. Seguin and his teachers also believed in "moral instruction." They saw themselves as more highly developed than the children they taught. Thus, they could impose their "superior" wills on their students. This attitude, though an improvement over shackles and abuse, was the beginning of the "do to" mentality that continues to this day. Teachers, therapists and social workers are thought to know what's good for the person who has trouble learning or getting along in the world. For many years peopled with disabilities have been treated, trained and tampered with "for their own good."

AMERICA'S TRAINING SCHOOLS

In 1848 Seguin moved to America. He wanted to bring his new ideas to the country that was, itself, a new idea. America was ripe for such a visit. In most small towns in the United States people who had mental disabilities or mental illness were free to roam about, usually protected by the townspeople who knew them. The "village idiot" was a creature who was tolerated, sometimes made fun of, sometimes taken advantage of. No one thought about sending people off somewhere to be treated.

If a person got into trouble, however, regardless of his mental abilities, he was put in prison. The prisons of the day were almost beyond anything we can imagine. Prisoners were beaten, chained, starved and left in the cold. And a person didn't have to commit a crime to be placed in a foul institution. If a woman couldn't take care of herself or her children, for whatever reason, she was sent to one of the almshouses erected for the care of "unfortunates." These places, too, were barely adequate to sustain life…not much better than Bedlam. Into this situation Seguin brought the new French approach that "feebleminded" people should be identified and segregated from others so that they could be educated and trained. People whose problems were seen as being the result of a disability rather than a moral failure would be given better treatment than the poor and the criminal.

At this time a teacher in a small town in Massachusetts, Hervey B. Wilbur became fascinated by the reports he read of Seguin's success with "idiot children" in France. He set up a school in his home in 1850. Several children at a time lived with Wilbur's family and were taught social graces and job skills so they could return to their homes as productive members of their society...rather than as "village idiots."

Soon other schools like Wilbur's were established in Pennsylvania, New York and Ohio. They were all small, homelike affairs with only a few students. The students lived like family and benefited from the individual attention and care they received.

There weren't enough small training schools for the thousands of people who needed them, though. Most still ended up in the prisons and poorhouses. This was the situation addressed by another Massachusetts reformer, Dorothea Dix. Dix was appalled by the living conditions she saw on her visits to prisons and poorhouses. She and another prison reformer, Samuel Gridley Howe, proposed the establishment of large public facilities for the humane care of "idiots, epileptics, and the insane." The proposal got much public support, but the Civil War came along and disrupted everyone's plans.

After the Civil War, there were lots of people wandering the roads looking for work, trying to put their lives back together. The graduates of the early training schools, who had learned enough skills to work productively in their home communities, were now not needed in the labor force.

Fortunately the public was now well aware that people who had mental disorders could be educated and trained. There was a call for the establishment of public institutions, and the first large, state-operated facilities were built. But the home environment and personal attention, so important for the success of the training schools, was lost in the larger setting. The state schools went back to being asylums, safe places for people with disabilities to be kept away from the rest of the community. Instead of training people to return home to work and community life, the custodial ("taking care of") institutions put them to work running the institutions themselves. Even as late as 1975, when I started to work at Colin Anderson Center there were still the remains of a working dairy farm and lumber mill. The people who lived in the institution raised the food, built the buildings and sometimes manufactured goods for sale on the outside. They were completely segregated from the rest of society.

At the same time as large training schools were being built, so too were large state hospitals for "the insane." They had doctors, rather than educators, in charge and were seen as more in line with the new scientific attitudes of the day. It wasn't long before the state schools jumped on the medical model bandwagon. They, too, began to have doctors as Superintendents. They began to separate residents on the basis of degree and type of disability—one "cottage" for "high grade morons" and another for "epileptics." The main concerns of the Superintendents were cleanliness, safety, and an orderly routine. Under this model, people with developmental disabilities were seen as in need of custodial care and productive work. They were not going to return to their home communities.

Though this era right after the Civil War might seem like ancient history, with no relevance to what you are doing today, look again. The establishment of the large, state operated facility was a model that has stayed with us even to the present day. Such facilities still keep people with disabilities separated from their home communities. They still have mandatory treatment (training) programs. They still have living units separated by functioning level, behavioral characteristics, or type of disability. As we continue our review of history, you will see many changes and improvements. But you will also see much that, unfortunately, has remained the same.

FEAR OF THE FEEBLEMINDED— THE RISE OF THE EUGENICS MOVEMENT

In 1906, two French educators, Alfred Binet (bin-AY) and Theodore Simon (see-MOAN), developed a test for French school children to determine which of them could benefit from public education and which could be sent to special schools. Binet warned that this test did not really measure any irreversible characteristic of the children.

The test was brought to America as the Binet-Simon test and later adapted by Louis Terman at Stanford University to become known as the Stanford-Binet. Terman called what was measured by the test "IQ" or "intelligence quotient." He claimed the IQ test was a real measure of a person's intellectual capacity, a capacity that was fixed for life and inherited from one's parents. Criminals and immigrants were given the new test and, sure enough, they turned out to be "intellectually deficient." People began to believe that the problems of society—crime, poverty, violence—were due to allowing so many intellectually substandard people to live and breed freely.

A new movement arose called "Eugenics," which means "well born." It was thought that if "mentally defective" people were locked in institutions and sterilized to keep them from breeding, society's problems would quickly go away.

This was no fringe movement of ill-tempered Nazi's. Many of the country's leading scholars, politicians and business leaders subscribed to the eugenics ideas. The whole sad era was symbolized by one case that was heard by the US Supreme Court in 1927. The case was known as Buck v. Bell. Bell, the defendant in the case, was the Superintendent of the Virginia State Colony for Epileptics and Feeble Minded. The plaintiff in the case was Carrie Buck, a woman who lived at the Virginia Colony. Court documents described Carrie Buck as:

> ...*a feeble-minded white woman who was committed to the State Colony for Epileptics and Feeble Minded. She is the daughter of a feeble-minded mother in the same institution, and the mother of an illegitimate feeble-minded child. She was eighteen years old at the time of the trial of her case in the Circuit Court in the latter part of 1924.*

Carrie Buck's complaint against Bell was that he ordered her to be sterilized against her will. The case worked its way to the US Supreme Court for a ruling on whether or not Carrie Buck's rights were violated. The Chief Justice at the time was the famous Oliver Wendell Holmes, a world renowned legal scholar. Holmes wrote the opinion of the Court:

> *The judgment finds the facts that have been recited and that Carrie Buck 'is the probable potential parent of socially inadequate offspring, likewise afflicted, that she may be sexually sterilized without detriment to her general health and that her welfare and that of society will be promoted by her sterilization,' and thereupon makes the order. We have seen more than once that the public welfare may call upon the best citizens for their lives. It would be strange if it could not call upon those who already sap the strength of the State for these lesser sacrifices,*

often not felt to be such by those concerned, in order to prevent our being swamped with incompetence. It is better for all the world, if instead of waiting to execute degenerate offspring for crime, or to let them starve for their imbecility, society can prevent those who are manifestly unfit from continuing their kind. Three generations of imbeciles are enough.

Social policy had run a course from a position of protecting people with disabilities from abuse and exploitation (giving asylum) to protecting society from what was known as "the menace of feeblemindedness."

NEGLECT AND WORSE

The years after Carrie Buck was seen as a menace to society were not an easy time for anyone. The Great Depression hit worldwide, bringing large scale unemployment and poverty. You can imagine that the conditions for people living in the large institutions also only got worse.

The Second World War brought two events that had a profound impact on treatment of people with disabilities. The first was the extermination by the Nazis of 100,000 "defectives," people who had mental retardation, cerebral palsy, and other disabilities. When eugenics had led simply to segregation in large facilities it didn't seem too bad. When it led to wholesale killing, it was shown up for the atrocity it was.

The second interesting event of the war was that there were many conscientious objectors who refused military service. Though they refused to fight, they were required to do community service. Many of them chose to work in the large state schools and hospitals. Their reports of the appalling conditions at those places raised people's awareness and paved the way for another wave of reform.

Another group that got organized to let society know what was going on was the parents of the people whose only option for care was the large state schools and hospitals. Parents had been told their children would never amount to anything and would have to be sent away. The parent groups that later became The Association of Retarded Citizens, now known as The Arc, took as their motto: "Retarded Children Can Be Helped!"

In 1964, the daily rate for caring for a person with a disability in an institution was about $5.57, half of what was spent at the time to keep an animal in a zoo. Indeed, some of the institutions would have been shut down if they had been zoos! They were dirty. The people living in them did not receive adequate food or clothing. There was nothing to do but sit around all day. Physical and psychological abuse was common.

While the parents were organizing and speaking out, other voices were being raised. 1966 saw the publication of *Christmas in Purgatory*, a photo essay that recorded the conditions at the large institutions. One of its authors, Burton Blatt, wrote, "there is a hell on earth, and in American there is a special inferno—the institution."

Senator Robert Kennedy visited Willowbrook State School in New York in 1965. One of his sisters had mental retardation. He described the place as "a snake pit." And in 1970 a young TV journalist returned to Willowbrook with cameras. His name was Geraldo Rivera, and his report brought more calls for reform.

All through these years of the 50's and 60's, there were two different approaches to fixing the problems everyone was becoming aware of. One approach was to try to reform the institutions, to clean them up and make them nicer places. The other approach, called "deinstitutionalization," wanted to shut down the large facilities and offer what became known as "community based services."

A FRESH BREEZE (ICF-MR)

The institutional reform movement won its most significant victory with the establishment in the mid-1970's of the ICF-MR section of the Medicaid program. ICF-MR stands for Intermediate Care Facility—Mental Retardation. "Intermediate" means "between one thing and another." In this case ICF-MR level of care fell between community based "day hospitalization" programs (with no residence) and Skilled Nursing Facilities (SNF), which provided intensive hospitalization for people who had serious medical needs. Under the new law, the Federal government told the states that if they would follow the rules put forth in the ICF-MR standards, the states would receive Federal Medicaid dollars to reimburse them for services to people with mental retardation. In other words, the money was there for states to make necessary reforms to their long-term care institutions.

Here's where the history I studied meets the history I lived. The ICF-MR standards came into being while I was working at 127 North Crib.

The problem for a place like Colin Anderson Center in 1977 was that the new standards meant a whole new way of doing things. The standards had radical requirements like "no more than four people to a bedroom" and "individualized treatment plan" and "clothes like those worn in the community." We never did anything like that on 127 North Crib.

So the Administration at Colin Anderson Center put together a plan to meet the strict requirements (and get the money). A new building was built that would meet ICF-MR standards. Called the "Modular Treatment Building" (or "mod building," for short), it was designed as six living areas that would each provide four bedrooms and a dayroom for 16 residents. Now, four people to a bedroom may not sound so great to you; but compared with the big wards, where 40 or more people slept in rows of beds, it was great!

We started a new program called ECHO ("Each Child Has Opportunity"), a program that provided individual assessments and training goals for each person in the program. ECHO residents had their own clothes (not the basic pullover shirts and elastic band pants that were made by volunteers in the Sewing Room.) They went to school and had speech therapy and recreational activities. They ate their meals family style in a dining room that was separate from the "living area." It was like a miracle.

The ICF-MR regulations were the cutting edge of institutional reform 25 years ago. Unfortunately, the rules haven't changed much since then.

"NORMALIZATION" AND "DEINSTITUTIONALIZATION"

Though the ICF-MR standards made the large state facilities more humane places to live, they still had problems. As we'll talk about in depth in the next chapter, there is an institutional attitude that is pretty much unavoidable when large groups of people with disabilities live together.

In 1972, Wolf Wolfensberger published a book called *The Principle of Normalization in Human Services*. He proposed that it is only in "normal" communities that people who have mental retardation will learn behaviors that will lead to social acceptance. This was called the principle of "normalization." Wolfensberger's ideas rallied a lot of support for closing down all large institutional facilities and helping people with disabilities return to their home communities. The process was known as "deinstitutionalization." In the 1980's, many states closed their large facilities and established "community based services."

During these years, landmark legislation was guiding the mental health field toward community based services. In 1963 President Lyndon Johnson signed the Developmentally Disabled Assistance and Bill of Rights Act. This law established such important ideas as a "right to treatment" and that people should receive treatment and support in the "least restrictive environment." The law was tested in the US Supreme Court in 1981 in the famous Pennhurst decision. The Court said it was, indeed, Congress' intent that people with disabilities have rights but that the states couldn't be forced to pay for their implementation. That's one that's still being argued today, as you'll see.

The Rehabilitation Act of 1973 required affirmative action programs for people with disabilities in businesses having Federal contracts and prohibited discrimination in services and employment by any agency or business that received Federal funds. It's been revised and renewed several times since then and is the basis of many of the training programs now available for people with disabilities.

One of the reasons parents had been supportive of institutional placements for their children who had disabilities was that they felt the institutions were the only place where there were adequate education and training services. A lot of kids with disabilities just stayed home from school. School systems told their parents, "We've got nothing for somebody like that." That began to change in 1975 with the passage of The Education for All Handicapped Children Act (PL94-142). This law requires that all children with disabilities should be granted a "free appropriate public education" in the least restrictive environment possible. It, too, has been revised, most recently in 1990, when it became known as IDEA (the Individuals with Disabilities Education Act). We'll talk more about how it works in Chapter 12—Disabilities Through the Lifecycle.

NEW LIFE IN THE NEIGHBORHOOD?

The most common model of support for those people who were moving out of the large institutions was the group home. Group homes had anywhere from three to ten people with disabilities living together in homes that were either built for the purpose or were purchased on the open market. Many of these homes were paid for by Medicaid and still followed the ICF-MR regulations. People who lived in group homes usually received clinical services from community mental health centers and got vocational and other training at regional sheltered workshops. In most cases, group home living was better than living on a ward, but there were problems. Many communities did not want group homes in their neighborhoods, so many of the group homes became isolated islands, cut off from community inclusion.

Other people who were "deinstitutionalized" ended up in nursing homes or on the streets. Some estimates suggest as many as 75% of the homeless people in our large cities may be people who have moved out of state facilities and are now receiving no support at all.

SELF-DETERMINATION AND THE OLMSTEAD DECISION

People continue to move out of large institutional facilities, but the pressure to move isn't coming from academic theories about what is "normal." This time, the pressure is coming from people who have learned to speak up for themselves and demand the kind of life they see as being free and dignified.

Many of the people I worked with in group homes began demanding more—more freedom, more opportunity, more control over their own lives. Once they'd had a taste of community life, of having jobs and friends and money in their pockets, they were no longer satisfied with being "placed" somewhere they didn't choose. They wanted to choose their own jobs, their own homes, their own roommates. They wanted to live real lives. We'll talk about this a lot more in Chapter 4—"Life Planning –Then and Now."

Recently the US Supreme Court has handed down a ruling that is causing a big stir through the states and the organizations that support people who have disabilities. Commonly known as the Olmstead Decision, the new ruling upholds the claims of two women (known as E.W.

and L.C. in the lawsuit) who lived in an institution in Georgia. The women claimed they had been asking for years for the opportunity to move to their own apartments in their home communities. They said the mental health professionals of Georgia had told them their moving would be "inappropriate." The court upheld their claim. It ruled that under the Americans with Disabilities Act (ADA) of 1991, the women were being discriminated against on the basis of their disability. E.W. and L.C. have moved out of the institution and have revealed themselves as Elaine Wilson and Lois Curtis. In a news conference celebrating their victory, Ms. Wilson said, "Now that I'm in the free world, I love my freedom. When I was in the hospital, I felt like I was in a little box, and I couldn't get out." Ms. Curtis added, "I just want to say the best thing is that now I get to go to my room and listen to my radio whenever I want."

PAST—PRESENT—FUTURE

We've come a long way since Bedlam. We've come a long way since Colin Anderson Center. We've even come a long way since deinstitutionalization and normalization. But we've still got a way to go. Throughout the rest of this book, you'll meet people who are pushing the envelope, insisting we move into the 21st century. And you'll have to think about issues that will affect the work you do every day. As you make this journey, don't forget where we've been. We've come a long way. But we've still got a long way to go.

Chapter 3

FROM INSTITUTION TO INCLUSION

In the last two chapters I have talked about places you would probably call "institutions"—Bedlam, Willowbrook, and the Colin Anderson Center where I first began this work. If you've visited or worked at one of these places you know that they are not like the scenes you grew up with or the neighborhoods you live and work in now.

What makes those places "institutions"? Is it that there are large brick buildings with long hallways? Is it that they are noisy and smell bad? Is it that they are run by bureaucrats and committees? Is it that lots of people live together? It's all of those things, for sure. Stepping into an institutional environment is like leaving the real world, the world we usually live in, and entering a fake world. The institutional world is made to seem like a place where someone would live, but it's not really so. And the lives that are lived there are not real lives like mine and yours. They are made up, pretend lives, scheduled, planned and organized. We know as soon as we walk into an institutional place that something is missing. We sense that the people who live there are missing some of the experiences and freedoms that we cherish in our own lives. We wouldn't want to live there.

I have worked in such unreal places for many years. I've known lots of good people who worked there and couldn't wait to get home to the "real world." And I've known many courageous people who've lived institutional lives and couldn't wait to get a "real life." That's why I say the most important thing you can do is to support what I call "Real Life in the Real World" for people with disabilities.

"INSTITUTION" IS AN ATTITUDE

Institutions are not places. They don't have signs out front saying *Welcome to The Institution.* In fact, I like to refer to "institutional environments" rather than to "institutions." It gives you more of the feeling that "institutional" describes a set of attitudes. "Institutional" is a way of doing things and a way of thinking about people.

Over the years, I've thought a lot about what makes a place or a program or a life "institutional." I think there are certain common characteristics of the institutional attitude toward people with disabilities. You can find these characteristics in big state-operated mental retardation facilities, as well as in nursing homes and group homes and day activity centers. But you can also find them in schools and supported living programs and supported employment. If the attitudes are there, the place is institutional. If they aren't, it's not.

So what makes a place institutional? I think the four most important characteristics are:

- Segregation
- People are put in labeled boxes
- Not enough attention
- Lack of control over your own life

SEGREGATION

You know how realtors say there are three important qualities for selling a home or business—location, location, location? Well, I'm tempted to say the same thing about the institutional attitude. The three most important characteristics are—segregation, segregation, segregation.

Segregation means "separation"—some group of people living in a world apart from others, with separate standards and separate goals. But segregation is more than simple separation. Segregation is also an injustice done to a minority group by the majority in power. Segregation means living on the reservation, in the ghetto, in the institution.

In American history, we are most familiar with the word segregation as it applied to the separation of people based on race. As a nation, we challenged the acceptability of such separation in the historic Brown v. Board of Education of Topeka, Kansas ruling by the Supreme Court in

1954. In that decision, the Court took the position that "separate" is always "unequal." Chief Justice Earl Warren wrote:

> *To separate [Negro children] from others of similar age and qualifications solely because of their race generates a feeling of inferiority as to their status in the community that may affect their hearts and minds in a way unlikely ever to be undone.... We conclude that in the field of public education the doctrine of "separate but equal" has no place. Separate educational facilities are inherently unequal.*

It was 20 years after that ruling before the same principle was applied to children who had disabilities (PL 94-142 — The Right to Education of All Handicapped Children Act of 1975). That law, which has been affirmed and renewed several times, said segregation of children with disabilities was as much a violation of their opportunities as was segregation because of race. The Right to Education of All Handicapped Children Act said that children with disabilities might also get "a feeling of inferiority as to their status in the community" if they were separated from everyone else.

But segregation in schools still exists. It's not based on race anymore. Instead, the segregation is based on intellectual ability. Children with disabilities are still educated in separate, "self-contained" classrooms, often in separate, "special" schools. They have little opportunity to get to know life in the real world and are being trained to accept a separate life, distant from many of the opportunities we take for granted. I call that institutional.

Adults with disabilities, too, are often placed in segregated environments. Sometimes these places don't seem like institutions. Indeed, they are usually called "community placements." But what if a person wakes up in the group home (which he shares with five other people with disabilities), rides the special van to the sheltered (segregated) workshop, then rides back to the group home for the night? He never gets a chance to interact with other people in the community. Isn't his life segregated?

We have seen that in the 1970's and 80's there was a great movement toward "deinstitutionalization." The federal government passed amendments to the Medicaid regulations that supported the development of

Home and Community Based Services (HCBS). Many states closed their large facilities (like Willowbrook and Colin Anderson Center). Thousands of people moved into small group (3-10 people) residences on streets in communities across the country. But were they really deinstitutionalized? Were they really reunited with the rest of society, or were they simply moved from a large segregated facility into a small one? Did the attitude that keeps people with disabilities in their place, separate from the mainstream, go away? I don't think so. I think we still have work to do to overcome the fact of segregation based on ability.

PREJUDICE AND FEAR

Segregation doesn't just harm its victims by denying them opportunity. Segregation of a minority group also makes them unknown to the majority. The segregated people are seen as "them," a group we never get to know because they live in a different, separate world. If we don't know people as individuals, we will only know what we've heard about the group. Our attitudes will be based on prejudice and fear, rather than on real relationships with real people.

When I was a child, growing up in the all white suburbs of Chicago, I was taught to be careful about the black people who lived in the inner city. I was warned that black people were violent and would probably rob me if I encountered them on the street. Now, that was a really stupid attitude. But why was I able to believe it? Because I grew up in a segregated world. Everyone in my world was just like me. I didn't know any black people as people, only as a feared group. Segregation had allowed me to be ignorant and fearful. And it cut me off from valuable relationships and opportunities for growth.

Most people have not had the opportunity to know someone with disabilities personally. All they know is stereotypes, usually negative.

One chilly fall evening, I found myself sitting at a long table in the Council meeting room of a small town in New Jersey. I was one of a group of professionals sent to the meeting by the company I worked for. We were supposed to answer any questions or objections the assembled citizens had to a proposed group residence the company was opening in one of the town's neighborhoods. I felt like I was sitting before a firing squad.

The people were angry and scared. They felt their neighborhood was being violated and that the lives of their children were in jeopardy.

Though the worried citizens had never met the three men who were going to live in the house, they each carried a vision of what "mentally retarded person" meant. It was a scary vision, like the one implanted in me about inner city people with dark skin. At one point I heard myself saying, "You people don't know who you're talking about. The guys who are moving in here are a little slow to learn, and they've been away at the state facility a long time. So they're going to need help integrating with your community. But I think you'll find that they can be great neighbors and even good friends."

I had the sinking feeling I was speaking a foreign language. Arms remained tightly crossed and faces were firmly set. I knew it was precisely *because* those guys had been segregated, moved away from their home towns, that nobody knew who they really were. But to the assembled crowd, they were mysterious strangers, probably convicts or child molesters. Segregation had done its deadly work on all concerned.

INTEGRATION

Integration, the bringing together of people who have lived separately, is a powerful antidote to this poisonous institutional attitude. Another word for integration is "inclusion." Inclusion means everyone is included in everything. No one is left out.

The US Developmental Disabilities Assistance and Bill of Rights Act is the law that tells what standards are to be upheld when Federal money is spent on disabilities services. It contains a description of what is meant by integration:

> *The term "integration and inclusion" with respect to individuals with developmental disabilities, means—*
>
> *(A) the use by individuals with developmental disabilities of the same community resources that are used by and available to other citizens;*
>
> *(B) living in homes close to community resources, with regular contact with citizens without disabilities in their communities;*
>
> *(C) the full and active participation by individuals with developmental disabilities in the same community activities and*

types of employment as citizens without disabilities, and utilization of the same community resources as citizens without disabilities, living, learning, working, and enjoying life in regular contact with citizens without disabilities; and

(D) having friendships and relationships with individuals and families of their own choosing.

These are the elements of Real Life in the Real World—the opportunity for all people, regardless of any personal characteristics that make them seem different, to work, play, and live together. We sacrifice this opportunity if we see people with disabilities as belonging in some separate community "for their own good."

As a direct support person, you can take an active role in breaking down the barriers of segregation. You can help the people you support meet their neighbors and start to be seen as a valuable addition to the neighborhood. You can help people make use of integrated community resources and stay away from the "special" events that are only for people with disabilities. You can help people establish networks of friends and coworkers who can open doors to full inclusion.

We must move beyond any "programs" or "services" which are not fully inclusive of everyone. We need to bring people together for the good of everyone.

PEOPLE PUT IN LABELED BOXES

Labels are the basis of segregation. Lloyd and Billy were moved from their homes to Colin Anderson Center not because they were Lloyd or Billy but because they were "retarded." We put them in the box, closed the lid and slapped a label on the side.

The institutional approach is full of labels. People are put into boxes labeled "high functioning" and "low functioning" or "ambulatory" and "non-ambulatory." The bad boxes are labeled "behavior disordered" (BD) or "behaviorally and emotionally handicapped" (BEH) or "high control." At Colin Anderson Center we had boxes for "Big Boys," "Big Girls," "Little Boys," and "Little Girls." You might think these were boxes for children, but it wasn't so. Everyone who lived in those wards (boxes) was an adult. The difference between Big Girls and Little Girls was that the Big Girls were large, aggressive adult women; and the Little Girls were small adult women who were more likely to be victimized.

The boxes of the institutional attitude are used as a management tool, for the convenience of staff. It's easier to train staff to deal with assaultive residents if they all live in the same place. You can get a teacher with specialized training and experience to deal with the "trainables" who are all boxed together in the self-contained classroom.

Sometimes the labels applied to people are called a "diagnosis" and are based on what we assume to be a scientific "assessment." We'll talk about diagnosis and assessment a lot more in later chapters. The important point here is that labels that put a person in a box by saying "That's all you are—no more, no less" keep us from seeing a lot of things about that person. It doesn't matter whether the label is applied by a doctor or by the guy on the corner. I am nearsighted and have to wear glasses. My diagnosis is "myopia." I sure wouldn't like it if people started saying, "Oh, yeah; I know James. He's that myope." Myopia isn't all there is to me. It's not even the most important thing about me. I don't want to be boxed in by my diagnosis. Likewise, a person who has mental retardation doesn't want to have to stay in a box marked "retarded." He probably doesn't even want to be in the box labeled "special." He doesn't want to be in the box at all. He wants to live a wide open life like you or me.

Sometimes professional people argue in favor of labels as a tool for deciding who gets a particular kind of support service. For example, a diagnosis of autism entitles a person to get services in the autistic class or live in the autistic group home. That seems like a good thing. Parents are told that such children have "special" needs that can only be met in a "special" (segregated) environment. The label entitles the person to the service. But how can you prepare someone to live in the world with the rest of us by isolating her from anyone who is not like her? Who is she going to learn from?

The problem with this isolation of people "for their own good" was elegantly stated by an elementary school student who was asked whether his classmate (who was labeled "autistic," "non-verbal," and "disruptive") should be in a separate class. His answer: "No; because if he was in a separate class, he wouldn't have any friends." Out of the mouths of babes.

NOT ENOUGH ATTENTION

In one of my previous incarnations I worked as a "Behaviorist." My job was to deal with "bad behavior." I was the one who was called in when Kathy had episodes of running around the group home throwing lamps and couch cushions, or when Andrew went into loud, disruptive spells of "cussing."

Since I'm not a psychologist and could therefore exercise my beginner's mind, I would respond to the calls from staff by asking, "Why do you think he/she is doing these things?" Many, many times the answer was, "I think she's just doing it for attention." I say "many, many times," because attention is something that is in short supply in institutional environments.

Imagine the six-person group home. There are two staff on duty. One of them is helping Gerald cook supper. The other is assisting Sally with her toileting. No one is paying attention to the other four people who live there. If one of those four people decides he wants attention, he has probably learned how to get it—cause a disturbance. Yell, bite yourself, slap your neighbor, knock the TV to the floor, pull the fire alarm. These are the ways people get attention in attention-starved (institutional) environments.

People with disabilities sometimes need more supportive attention than people who can do things more on their own. Just ask a mother of a child with a disability. She'll tell you her son who has mental retardation and cerebral palsy needs a lot more attention than her other two typical kids. That's because he needs help with things.

Of course, there's nothing wrong with needing help and support. We all need it in various ways. And we have all learned various ways to get the attention we need. But if someone puts you in an institutional environment, in a large group, the rules change. The ways things work in an institutional place is like the crazy rules of a dysfunctional family. There's not enough attention to go around. The paid staff are often distracted by their own issues, or they've been told by their bosses that what's really important is stuff like documentation, scheduling, following safety rules, and cleaning (all those things I learned in Basic Aide training). Your need for attention gets lost in the shuffle.

Some people who don't get enough attention withdraw into a shell. You see them in institutional places, rocking, humming to themselves, waving their hands in front of their faces. This is called "stereotypical behavior" or "self stim"—repetitive, purposeless activities that make something happen, that reassure me I'm still here. I used to think people engaged in stereotypical behavior because they had mental retardation. I thought it was a symptom of their brain condition. But then I noticed that other people who live in institutions, people who don't get enough attention, act that way, too. People in understaffed nursing homes or psychiatric hospitals also rock and moan and cry out. They don't get enough attention.

Instead of withdrawing, some people take a different approach. They raise a ruckus. They pitch destructive tantrums, destroying property or hurting other people and themselves. They get attention for acting that way. Staff drop what they're doing and come running when someone starts tearing up the place. When there's not enough attention, you'll take what you can get—even the apparently negative attention of being held down on the floor, tied to your bed or locked in seclusion.

For more about how institutional lack of attention causes behavior problems, see Chapter 9, "Why Does She Act That Way?"

LACK OF CONTROL OVER YOUR OWN LIFE

I was once called to one of the group homes because Ted had "pitched a fit" the night before. He had torn up his bedroom, punched a staff person, and kept everyone up until after midnight. Why had he acted that way? Because in the middle of a play-off basketball game on TV, the staff had told him he had to go to bed. It was 9:00 PM. Ted was 26 years old.

Ted's response made sense to me. I asked the staff why they thought they needed to send him to bed at 9:00. They answered, "If he stays up late, he'll be tired at work." Well, sure; that would be the case with me, too. The difference is that I get to decide whether it's more important to me to watch the big game than it is to be rested at work. I have control over many facets of my life. Ted doesn't.

So what was Ted saying when he pitched his tantrum (staying up well past "bedtime" you may have noticed)? The actual words that came out of his mouth were threats and curses that can't be repeated here. But what he was communicating was, "Leave me alone and let me run my own life!" Seems a reasonable request from an adult man. But the institutional attitude won't let it happen. Why not?

There are a number of reasons. The first and most obvious reason is that most institutional environments have large groups of people. When you're trying to manage a large group, individuals lose control. After all, you can't have everybody running off in a different direction trying to run their own life, can you? Everyone has to follow rules that are designed for the smooth operation of the facility.

Another reason for institutional control over people's lives is the belief that if people with disabilities are allowed to make decisions for themselves, they will make bad choices. They will choose unwisely and make mistakes. Sound like anyone you know? Yourself maybe? Me, too. I've made tons of mistakes in my life, sometimes the same one repeatedly. But no one ever told me they were going to take away my right to run my life in my own muddled, crazy way. I wouldn't have let them. I would have pitched a fit.

This reason for taking away the right of people with disabilities to control their own lives becomes a self-fulfilling prophecy—because we act like it's true, it comes true. When we don't let people run their own lives, sure enough, they never learn how to run their own lives. See, we were right about them all along.

The way you learn to make good decisions is by making decisions and learning from what happens. Institutional control takes away that opportunity, and people get stuck, seen as lifelong children, not even able to decide when they want to go to bed.

The final, and most complicated, reason institutions take away control of people's lives is the matter of who's responsible for what happens. If I'm in charge of an institutional place and something bad happens to someone, guess who gets in trouble. Yeah, me. After all, the people in my care were put there because we believe they cannot be responsible for themselves.

If I'm responsible for what happens to you, am I going to let you make mistakes that might have bad consequences? Of course not. I'm going to protect you from those consequences by making the "right" decisions for you. I take away your rights "for your own good."

This issue of responsibility and how it relates to rights can get very tricky. It's one of the reasons this institutional attitude is still so common. For more on this issue, see Chapter 11, "Sex, Smokes and the Responsible Adult."

Chapter 3 – From Institution to Inclusion

WHY DOES THIS MATTER?

There you have, in a nutshell, the characteristics, the attitudes, that I think make a place an institution. Institutions separate people from the mainstream of society, into boxes with labels, where they don't get enough attention and don't have control over their own lives.

Why should this matter to you? The place where you work isn't an institution, is it? Well, maybe it has some of the characteristics. Maybe it has all of them. What can you do about it? That's a lot of what this book is about. I've worked many years in places that violated people's rights and treated people badly. I didn't like a lot of what I saw. But at every one of those places, there were people with good hearts and good values who also didn't like it. Together we could make a difference. *We* are the staff. *We* make the environment. *We* are the ones who either empower people with disabilities or treat them with disrespect and disregard. The institution is not a place; it is us. We can't blow it up or close it down, because it doesn't exist "out there." Rather, it is the attitudes we bring to our work. Together, we can make a difference. How? Let's look at some ways.

OUR STANDARD

A co-worker of mine once gave me a tool to hang in my office. It was a heavy metal weight, pointed at the bottom, hanging from a string—a plumb bob. Carpenters use them to make sure the walls they build are truly vertical. A strange gift, you might think. Why would she give me, a person who works to provide support for people with disabilities, a carpenter's tool? She said she wanted me to have it so that I would always remember to be true to "Our Standard." I had taught her that Standard when we first started to work together. And the plumb bob is still hanging right there on the wall as I write.

What is this Standard she was talking about? What is the line that tells us whether our supports are straight and true? Well, it's surely not something anybody learned in college. Nor is it a company policy decided by a committee in a board room. In fact, the tool I challenge you to take as your Standard in this work is not an answer, but a question, a question you need constantly to ask yourself—*Is this the kind of life I would like to live?*

31

Notice that I don't ask "Is this the kind of life I would like to live...if I had mental retardation?" or "Is this the kind of life I would like to live...if I had a disability?" No; we each have to ask, from our own personal values, "Is this the kind of life I would like to live?" Would I like to have someone telling me what time I have to go to bed at night, what I have to eat for supper, who I need to live with, where I need to live, what kind of job I need to have, who I should have as my friends, what my goals in life should be? I don't think so. Neither would you. And neither would the people you support.

When we use our own values and attitudes about life as Our Standard, we are affirming the basic principle of "Real Life in the Real World"— people with support needs are not so different from us that they need a different kind of life or have different kinds of personal goals and life dreams. The people we support are very much like you and me—they want to get ahead in life; they want to be somebody; they want to be loved and accepted; they want to feel valuable and needed.

So, if you're doing something, someday, in the name of "training" or "treatment" and you start thinking, "This is really stupid. *I* wouldn't want to do this," remember Our Standard...and think of a better way.

Another good thing about taking "Is this the kind of life I would like to live?" as Our Standard is that you don't need any special training to apply it. You don't need a degree in psychology or social work to ask yourself the question. All you need is a good heart, a willingness to see people with disabilities as being just as valuable and important as you are...and maybe a little familiarity with the Golden Rule. Treat other people the way you would want to be treated.

Once you get used to using your feelings as the Standard, you can move a step further. You can identify with the feelings of the person you support. It's called "empathy." Once you can really get to know that person and what's inside his heart, you can change Our Standard to, "Is this the kind of life the person I support wants to live?"

OUR LANGUAGE

The language you use when talking about people tells me a lot about what your attitude is toward those people. If you use terms of respect and appreciation, I know your attitude is positive. I can tell by the kinds of words you use that the people you are talking about are your loved ones or colleagues or friends.

If, however, you describe people using different words from those you use with your friends and family members, I'll know that you think of those people as being different. I'll know that you see them in some other category from your own group. I'll know that you see some people as "Us" and others as "Them."

"SPECIAL" WORDS FOR "SPECIAL" PEOPLE?

There are lots of technical terms in any field. These are special words that refer to the objects or techniques of a particular job. If you're a physical therapist, for example, you'll understand terms like "abduction," "adduction," and "flexion." They are specialized words that help those who use them communicate with others in their profession.

The field of support services for people who have disabilities is no different. We do have a lot of specialized terms. Just glance at the Glossary in the back of this book, and you'll see that. But in support services we're not only dealing with techniques and objects—we're dealing with people. And since we often think of the people we work with as "special," we will think it's OK to use "special" language with them.

But be careful! "Special" has too often been used to separate people, to put them in boxes that can then be set outside of Real Life in the Real World. When we refer to "Special Education," we are too often talking of segregated classes and sub-standard programs. When we talk about "Special Olympics," we are referring to a group of people we know are not part of the "real" Olympics. Calling it "special" is a way to justify the fact that it is separate and unequal. Does this kind of segregation meet Our Standard? Would we like to be put in a box marked "Special"?

UNIVERSAL LANGUAGE

Real Life in the Real World means everyone is included. We can't put people with support needs into separate worlds and lives. The way to stay honest with this is to make sure that you always use "Universal Language."

What is Universal Language? Well, it's language that is "universal," that is, "applied to everyone." The definition is easy to learn and easy

33

to apply: *Universal Language is the language we use with our family and friends and that they use with us.*

Has your mother ever referred to you as "high functioning"? No? Does that mean that you're "low functioning"? Maybe it means that "high functioning" and "low functioning" are not Universal Language terms, not the kind of thing your mother would say. She might say that you're "smart," "capable," "competent"—but she wouldn't say, "high functioning." "High functioning" is a "special" term that we only use with "them."

Think about it. Especially if you've worked in the disabilities field for awhile, you may have gotten used to applying terms to "them" that no one in your family or circle of friends would apply to anyone they considered a real person. Is your spouse, for example, ever "non-compliant?" Is that the term you use? "Honey, sometimes you're so non-compliant, I can't stand it!" And when you take your sweetheart to dinner on Friday night, do you call it an "outing?" When your brother helped haul your furniture to that new apartment, did you call it "being admitted?" And will you be "discharged" if you decide to live somewhere else?

One of the nice things about using Universal Language is that you don't have to learn any new terms. In fact, that's just the point—you use the same language with and toward people with disabilities that you already know and use with the people in your community.

PEOPLE FIRST

One form of language that has been around in our field for a fairly long time is "People First" language. It's as easy to learn and apply as Universal Language. You simply remember that people with disabilities are people first—and their disability comes later. For instance, we say "a person *with* mental retardation" rather than "a *mentally retarded* person." When you think about "a mentally retarded person," with the "person" part last, you think of a stereotype, somebody who is a faceless member of a group that you think you know something about. "Oh, yeah, 'retarded person'—somebody who can't do things, is weird, and maybe should be kept away from my kids." A "person *with* mental retardation," on the other hand, could also be a person with a good sense of humor, with a job at the local muffler shop, or with a fiancé.

Using People First language helps us remember that a disability is only one part of a person, and maybe not the most significant part.

WHAT TO CALL "THEM"

There is a great deal of discussion in the support services field about what to call "Them." We have gone through many fads, each of which was the "correct" term at the time.

When we kept people with developmental disabilities in the hospital, as if they had a long-term disease, we called them "patients."

When we thought the most important part of them was that they lived in the residences we provided for them, we call them "residents."

When we decided that the important thing about them was that they received professional services from us, we switched to "clients."

Recently, we have decided that the most important thing to remember is that they are paying the bills; so we have taken to calling them "consumers."

Lately, a new code word is creeping into people's speech—"individuals." I realized this new one was a code word for "Them" when I read in a newsletter that "two staff and five individuals had a good time on a picnic." If each "individual" ate three hot dogs, would they then become "consumers?"

All of the terms used above are perfectly good descriptions of roles we all occupy at one time or another. We are "patients" when we go to see our doctors. We are "residents" of the apartment complex where we live. We are "clients" of our hairdresser or lawyer or therapist. We are "consumers" when we grab our Visa card and head for Wal-Mart. And we're surely all proud to be "individuals."

Because we are "Us" and not "Them," we don't feel the need to pick one term to stand for who we are. We can move freely from role to role; and the fact that we are allowed to occupy many different roles is an important indicator that we are fully included members of our community.

The point is that no matter what the politically correct term of the month is, any term that serves to segregate people rather than include them demonstrates our non-inclusive attitudes. The point is to get rid of the divisions altogether.

So what would I like you to call "Them?" I'd like you to call them "people," as in "People (not "consumers") should have work that is rewarding." Or use their name, as in, "Sam (not "my client") is very proud of his new job."

Using Universal Language or People First Language or calling the person we work with by his name are not just new rules for the same old behavior. The words we use are important because they reflect our attitude about the people we work with; and attitude, as we all know, is the wellspring of behavior.

FROM INSTITUTION TO SELF-DETERMINATION

In this chapter we have seen how institutional attitudes keep people with disabilities from living a Real Life in the Real World. We have seen how our attitudes, our language, and our behavior can be used to resist institutional conditions. And we have seen that segregation, the most common institutional characteristic, can be dealt with through inclusion. Another of the institutional characteristics we have looked at is the fact that people who live in institutional environments have not had control over their own lives. That's beginning to change. We are coming into the era of self-determination. Let's take a closer look.

Chapter 4

LIFE PLANNING— THEN AND NOW

LIFE PLANNING

Some people are planners; some are not. There are people who seem to wander through life, grabbing opportunity as it comes. And there are people who have a plan for next week, next year, five years, and ten years.

Planners maintain there's no way to reach your goal unless the path is laid out clearly in front of you. Non-planners say, "Good luck is nothing but being ready to open the door when opportunity knocks."

These differences in how to move into the future will probably always be with us. But I can tell you one thing for sure—if you receive support services because of a disability, you certainly have a plan. Habilitation plans, treatment plans, transition plans, individualized education plans, behavior plans—these are everywhere in the disabilities support field. I've worked in some programs where it seemed we spent half our time planning what to do with the other half.

THE ICF-MR PLANNING MODEL

Plans came to us with the ICF-MR regulations of the 1970's. There were two reasons for plans being required by those new regulations. The first was that, until the regulations came to places like Colin Anderson Center, there were no plans of any kind. Everything was chaotic, repetitive, going nowhere.

The second reason was that ICF-MR is a medical model of services. In medicine, they have treatment plans, nursing plans, discharge plans. Medicine is seen as a clear road with a beginning (admission), a middle (treatment), and an end (discharge). A plan helps you get down that road.

The ICF-MR planning process is still used in many places. Many of the group homes that were established as part of deinstitutionalization still operate under the ICF-MR standards. This type of planning has become a standard in our field, and you need to know how it works. File it under "What We Have Done" and "What We Are (Still) Doing." It's not the best way to help people plan, and I'll show you some newer systems before the end of this chapter. For now, let's go through the standard planning process for a man named Wilbur. As we go through each step, try to spot areas you think could be done better.

ASSESSMENT

The planning process starts with an assessment of Wilbur's "current level of functioning." That means measuring and analyzing what Wilbur can and cannot do.

Starting with an assessment makes sense. You have to know where you are before you can decide where you want to go. In the ICF-MR system, assessments are done by clinical professionals from various disciplines (a discipline is a course of study, like nursing, social work, physical therapy, psychology). A clinician from each discipline will assess Wilbur's "strengths and needs." These are usually listed in two columns or two sections.

The social worker, for example, may list Wilbur's strengths as:
- Good family support
- Friendly and outgoing

She will then list Wilbur's needs. These might include:
- Cannot dial phone to call parents
- Greets strangers inappropriately
- Touches females inappropriately

Next, the nurse does a nursing assessment. On her report, Wilbur's only strength is listed as:
- Good general health

Under nursing needs, the nurse lists:
- Poor oral hygiene
- Does not wipe well after toileting
- Cannot administer medication
- 10 pounds over ideal body weight
- High cholesterol

All the clinicians on what is called the "interdisciplinary team" (because they come from different disciplines) write their assessments of Wilbur. Sometimes a licensed clinician will administer tests to get some standard measurement of Wilbur's functioning. The psychologist would probably give an IQ test. The physical therapist might test range of motion and upper body strength. The nurse might see that Wilbur gets an annual physical exam.

THE QMRP AND THE INTERDISCIPLINARY TEAM

Every team has to have a leader, and the ICF-MR interdisciplinary team is no exception. The leader of the team is a "QMRP" (Qualified Mental Retardation Professional), commonly referred to as "the Q."

All services paid for by Medicaid must be overseen by a Q. In addition to the QMRP, there are QDDP's (Qualified Developmental Disabilities Professionals), QMHP's (Qualified Mental Health Professionals), and QSAP's (Qualified Substance Abuse Professionals). The Q always stands for "Qualified," and the P stands for "Professional," and the letters in between stand for the type of disabilities the Q is qualified to oversee. In the Medicaid system the qualifications for Q status are written into the regulations. They require a four-year college degree and some number of years of supervised experience with the particular kind of disability.

The Q, as I said, is the head of the interdisciplinary team. She calls the team together for an annual planning meeting. She writes the plan. She has to review the plan to see if progress is being made toward the goals. If no progress is being made, she has to figure out why and make adjustments.

THE ANNUAL PLANNING MEETING

Back to Wilbur's plan. It's time for his annual planning meeting (required by the ICF-MR regulations). The Q has scheduled it several months in advance. Since all of the interdisciplinary team members are required to attend annual planning meetings, and each of them has 30 or more people on their case load, scheduling is often a problem. The meeting will be held next Thursday afternoon at 2:30 at the group home where Wilbur lives. Wilbur's mother is taking the day off of work so she can be there. Wilbur is going to be brought back from the workshop so he can participate.

Finally, the big day is here. The interdisciplinary team members arrive with their briefcases. Some of them inform the Q that they'd like to go first because they have other meetings to attend. In addition to the assessment reports, each team member also has suggestions for goals for Wilbur for the coming year. The ones who have to leave early will submit their goal recommendations in writing before they go.

When everyone is present, there are eight professional people sitting around the kitchen table with Wilbur and his mother—the Q, psychologist, nurse, social worker, physical therapist, speech language therapist, recreational therapist and vocational specialist. If you are a direct support staff person who works with Wilbur, you *might* be there, too. Everyone signs an attendance sheet as documentation that they were present.

The Q introduces everyone around the table and the reports are read. After the third report, Wilbur gets bored and starts pulling on his Mom's arm to get her to take him outside. The Q says, "Wilbur, this is your meeting. But it's your choice if you want to stay or not." Wilbur, who's played this game before, says, "Go outside." The Q turns to you and asks if you'd take Wilbur out to the patio. You're grateful for the distraction, because you were getting bored listening to the reports too.

While you and Wilbur are outside enjoying the sunshine (and you're sneaking a smoke), the Q and the team finish giving their reports and making their recommendations.

Remember the social worker from earlier? Her goals for Wilbur are:
1. By March 1, Wilbur will independently use the phone to call his parents.
2. By June 1, Wilbur will greet strangers appropriately 80% of the time for two consecutive weeks.
3. By June 1, Wilbur will have two consecutive weeks with zero incidents of touching females inappropriately.

Did you notice how the list has a goal for each of the needs listed in the social work assessment?

The nurse has her list of goals, too. Not surprisingly, her goals also tie in with the list of needs she came up with on Wilbur's assessment. Setting goals that address a person's needs is one of the requirements of the ICF-MR system. The nurse's goals are:

1. By March 1, Wilbur will have a complete dental check-up with follow-up visits for treatment as needed.
2. By October 1, Wilbur will brush his teeth adequately with minimal staff supervision.
3. By December 1, Wilbur will clean himself adequately after toileting for two consecutive weeks.
4. Wilbur's medications will be administered by a person properly credentialed to administer medication.
5. Wilbur will be placed on a low fat, heart healthy diet (no treats; no seconds) until he loses ten pounds and his cholesterol is within normal limits.

When everyone is done with their reports and their recommendations, the Q asks Mom if she has anything to add. Mom, who is thoroughly intimidated by all of these educated professionals and certainly doesn't want to say anything that would threaten Wilbur's placement at the group home, says, "No, you people are doing a fine job. I'm so glad Wilbur has people like you to take care of his needs. I'm very grateful to all of you."

Everyone rushes off to the next meeting, leaving you to deal with Wilbur, who is crying and yelling because his Mom left.

THE PLAN

The Q now has a stack of papers and notes that she has to turn into an acceptable Habilitation Plan for Wilbur. She will write out all of the approved goals. In the process she will make sure each goal meets the requirement that it be "measurable and time limited." "Measurable" means there has to be some way of knowing whether Wilbur is making progress toward the goal. The Q is the one who is going to have to write progress reports. And "time limited" just means you can't take forever (like we used to do) to work on a goal. She will then have to write a training program to go with each goal. The training program will have detailed instructions on how to train each task. That's so you and your colleagues will all train Wilbur the same way. The training programs will also have a documentation plan telling you how to keep track of how Wilbur is doing. The Q will use the documentation sheets to "assess progress," which is part of her job.

The Q also has to be sure Wilbur's plan is "individualized," that it's not the same as everyone else's plan. Of course, it won't be completely individualized, because the Q has a bunch of these plans to write. So she has a template in her word processor. She just fills in the blanks and voila!—an individualized habilitation plan for Wilbur has been accomplished for another year.

WHAT'S WRONG WITH THIS PICTURE?

The scenario we just went through is a typical presentation of the kind of planning that goes on for people with disabilities every day. It's not the best way; but it's very common. It's a system that has developed over the years to meet various requirements of regulations and limited staff and limited time. It has become "the way we do it." It's the box we usually think in. But a lot of people are thinking outside this box these days. If you're new to this field, you've got the advantage of never having been in the box in the first place. You can look at the situation with new eyes. You can apply Our Standard—"Is this the kind of life I would like to live?"

So look at Wilbur's planning process from outside the box. Look at it as if it is one of those pictures where you have to "find the five mistakes." What's wrong with this picture?

I hope you saw that the most obvious problem is that the Q and her team are in charge of the process. It's their meeting and their plan.

Who should be in charge? Of course, Wilbur—with the help of his Mom, if he wants it. Sure, they were invited to the meeting. But they had to change their usual plans to meet the schedule needs of the team. That makes it clear whose meeting it really is.

One of the battle cries of the self-advocacy movement has been "nothing about us without us." Don't talk about our problems, our needs, our bad behaviors without us being present to speak up for ourselves. A planning session without the active participation of the person whose plan it is is a professional lie.

In order for Wilbur to be in charge of his planning meeting, what would we have to do? Well, first the professionals would have to step aside. Remember how in the institutional approach support provider agencies take responsibility for the people they support? In the ICF-MR system, it's the professionals who are held responsible by the system. They must do the planning on time, in the correct way, with all the appropriate signatures. They could lose their licenses if they perform badly. Naturally, they want to be in charge. But it's Wilbur's life that's at stake here. He and his Mom and anyone else in their supportive circle of friends and family should be calling the professionals to his meeting, at a time and place that are convenient to them. We work for the people we support; they don't work for us.

Next, we'd have to actually get to know Wilbur. That's another mistake in the current picture. Right now all we know is that he doesn't wipe well and that if you're a female staff person you'd better watch his hands. None of the professional assessments gave us an idea of who Wilbur is. We never really met him. He seems like just some retarded guy who lives in a group home. Could you imagine someone making a plan for your life if she didn't even know who you really are? You'd want your life plan to be based on your dreams and desires and what you want to be when you grow up. You'd want the plan to help you overcome your fears. You'd want a plan that recognizes your gifts and helps you overcome your gaps. You'd want people who really know you and care about you to help you make your plan. Wilbur wants no less.

Another "mistake" in this picture is that it's all inside the box that is support services for people with disabilities. Did you notice that the social worker referred to Wilbur's behavior as "inappropriate"? What does that mean? It's just a leftover from the institutional approach where we wanted to get rid of "inappropriate" behavior and replace it with "appropriate" behavior. It really says nothing about Wilbur's life goals and what kinds of support he might need to reach them.

The assessments came up with the same old "needs." The goals can be met by using the same old training programs. It's all the same old same old. Wilbur's Mom is satisfied with it because it seems to be the best the system has to offer. Wilbur isn't satisfied with it, but he can't really express that, and no one wants to hear it.

Finally, the goals that are recommended are doomed to failure. Why? Because they didn't come from Wilbur. I suspect Wilbur doesn't really care about his weight or his cholesterol level. He probably doesn't even care about his messy pants. If Wilbur doesn't care about his goals, and you're supposed to make sure he achieves them, what we end up with is a power struggle. And in a power struggle—everybody loses.

The planning game, as practiced every day in hundreds of places across the country, is tired and worn out. It wastes a lot of time and other resources. It needs to be replaced. Fortunately, there are better ways.

PERSON-CENTERED PLANNING

"Person-centered" has been a buzz word in disabilities services for the last decade or more. No matter whether the planning process is modeled after the medical treatment plan or revolves around the work of an interdisciplinary team, the plan that results has always been assumed to be "person-centered." That means all of the work that goes into the plan should center on the person for whom the plan is being developed. That makes sense, doesn't it? If it's my plan, I want it to be centered on me.

We have seen, though, how thinking inside the box has gotten us into bad habits. Too often "person-centered" is thought of as a particular part of the planning process, rather than the focus of all we do. We might say the plan is "person-centered" because we invited Wilbur to his planning meeting. He just didn't want to stay. We asked his Mom what she thought, and she said we were doing great. Wasn't that person-centered? Wasn't it individualized? Well, no; it wasn't. We didn't really take the time to get to know Wilbur and his needs. The professionals focused on their need to get their work done in a timely fashion. They paid most of their attention to the requirements of the regulatory agencies that provide the money. Mom focused on her need to have a safe place for Wilbur to live, so she can get on with her own life and that of her other three children.

And Wilbur just lives in the moment. He knows that right now he'd rather be outside than sitting in a meeting where people are talking about stuff he doesn't understand. He knows he's glad Mom's here, and he hopes she'll take him home with her. And he knows he likes being with you. You don't hassle him, and you're patient when he tries to tell you something.

What Wilbur doesn't know is what the possibilities are for him to have a life. He doesn't ask about having a job because he doesn't know what kind of job he could do. Nor does he know that having a job would bring him money that he could use to buy stuff that the group home people couldn't take away. And he doesn't know that Deirdre, the girl who works across the table from him at the workshop thinks he's pretty cute.

It turns out that our planning hasn't been person centered—it's been disability centered. We see it as our job to fix Wilbur's disability. We're trained to do that. Some of us have licenses that let us work on specific disabilities. We have become so wrapped up in the medical model (which is based on curing someone who is sick) that we've forgotten the person altogether. Our assessments ask the wrong questions of the wrong people.

What questions should we ask? Who should ask the questions? And who should we ask? How do we find out what Wilbur really wants and needs? How do we come up with a plan that efficiently guides our efforts in supporting Wilbur to have a real life in the real world? That's a lot of questions. It's a beginner's mind thing.

One of the strongest advocates for truly person-centered planning is Michael Smull (see Additional Resources for contact information). He has developed an approach to planning that is called "Essential Lifestyle Planning" (ELP), and it's an example of the excellent thinking that's getting us all out of the box. Michael gives a simple definition of what must be included in truly person-centered planning. He writes, "Good person-centered planning requires that you be able to learn what is important to each person, separate what is important to the person from what is important to others, and communicate what you have learned in a way that others understand." ("A Plan is not an outcome," 1998)

WHAT PEOPLE LIKE AND ADMIRE—GIFTS

Everyone has gifts, things he's good at and that people admire. That's why a good Essential Lifestyle Plan for Wilbur would start out with "What People Like and Admire About Wilbur."

We all want to be liked and admired, don't we? Do you think people would like and admire you because you can "toilet independently" or "have complete range of motion in upper extremities?" Hardly. People like and admire you because of your gifts, because you have a good sense of humor or are a good listener or are always willing to help. It turns out our friend Wilbur has a laugh that makes others feel good. And he has a way with animals and small children. They approach him because he's calm and gentle. You would never know these things from the "strengths" section of Wilbur's ICF-MR style plan.

How do we know these things about Wilbur? Can we administer a "gifts assessment?" Of course not. We ask the people who like to be around him—people who think he's a good guy.

WHAT WILBUR MUST HAVE IN HIS LIFE— DREAMS AND DESIRES

The next step is learning what is important to Wilbur. That wasn't included in the ICF-MR plan either. Instead of what's important to Wilbur, the assessments emphasized what's wrong with him.

We all have some things in life that are so important to us that they are a "must have." These are the things that give our life meaning. Without them we would be unhappy, frustrated, maybe even angry. For me, I "must have": the opportunity to do good work; intellectual stimulation through conversation or reading; and private time with my mate, time when I'm not "on." If someone took those things away from me, locked me up, took away my books, and prevented contact with my loved ones, I think I'd become very mean and withdrawn.

I've just told you what I must have in my life. I'm a word guy, so telling comes easily. But what about Wilbur? He doesn't use words. How do we know what he must have in his life? It can be summed up in two words—pay attention. Wilbur's behavior communicates how he feels about things. Listen. When he gets what he needs he has a "good day"; when he doesn't, he has a "bad day." By paying attention, you could make a list of the things that would make a good day for Wilbur and those that would make a bad day. For practice, try making such a list for yourself. You'll get a clear idea of what your own "must have's" are.

Those who know him well know that if Wilbur starts jumping up and down and biting the side of his hand things are not well with him. Something is wrong. Pay attention to these outbursts (and to the calm times) and you will see that Wilbur must have his room "just so." Don't mess with his stuff.

And he needs to see Mom at least once a week. He doesn't know what a week is, but he'll let you know if it's been too long between visits. He calls Mom on the phone every evening. He needs help pushing the buttons but he can hold the phone on his own. He doesn't talk, but he listens to Mom as she tells him about her day. He laughs a lot. Mom always limits the call to five minutes, and Wilbur has no problem with that.

Wilbur also wants a close physical relationship with a woman (not his mother) who cares about him. How do you know that? You've paid attention to the way he hugs and fondles female staff who are gentle with him. The social worker called it "inappropriate" and wanted to put him on a program to "decrease the frequency of the behavior." But you've also noticed how he lights up when he's with Deirdre at the workshop. You saw them holding hands under the work table.

Finally, Wilbur is a slow riser in the morning. He needs time to wake up gradually. He likes to sit in his underwear at the dining room table, have a cup of coffee and watch "Good Morning America" (he thinks Diane Sawyer looks like his Mom). He'll gladly brush his teeth later. This is what we call a "personal ritual." It's the way Wilbur has to start his morning in order to have a good day. What are your personal rituals? How would you feel if your boss came into your home and disrupted them?

Next on Wilbur's Essential Lifestyle Plan, we list his "likes and dislikes." These are the little choices and preferences we all make everyday. If we don't pay attention to Wilbur's preferences, we'll be running an institution, denying him choice.

It's amazing how many choices we express during a typical day. I take it for granted that I can use Arm & Hammer PeroxiCare Tartar Control toothpaste (I don't like mint gels) on my Oral B A-40 toothbrush (medium bristles). I shave with a Gillette Sensor Excel razor and Kiss My Face Natural Moisture Shave (Virgin Forest scent). I would not be a happy camper if I was placed somewhere where they made me use an electric toothbrush with soft bristles (because the dentist ordered it) and mint Crest toothpaste (yuck!). Try to train me to use an electric razor and I will be non-compliant. I don't like them.

Wilbur has strong likes and dislikes, too. We need to list them in his plan so everyone who works with him can honor his preferences. The list should include how he likes to be touched, how he likes to be talked to (and not talked to), what he likes to eat at each meal, what places he likes to go to, and what he likes to do there, who he likes to hang out with and who he doesn't want around. This is a plan for Wilbur to have the kind of life he wants. Honoring his preferences every day will go a long way toward making his life meaningful and satisfying and putting him in charge.

IN ORDER TO SUPPORT...

Have you noticed how this Essential Lifestyle Plan is truly centered on Wilbur? So far, we haven't prescribed any training programs for him. That's because the intent of this plan is not to "fix" Wilbur but to support him. The next section deals not with what we want Wilbur to do in the coming year but with what we need to do to support him. The goals are for us, in a section called "In Order to Support."

In order to support Wilbur, we first need to know how to communicate with him. Because Wilbur doesn't use words for communication, his new plan includes a section that puts down all the things we who know and work with Wilbur understand that he means by certain actions in certain situations. We make a chart with columns for: "When this is happening" (while he is eating, for instance); "And Wilbur does" (puffs air out through his lips and waves his hand rapidly in front of his mouth); "We think it means" (the food's too hot); "Then we should" (show him how to blow on the food to cool it down). Wilbur's communication chart is several pages long. It's a real help to people who are new to working with Wilbur. It assures Wilbur will always be treated in an understanding way that is respectful of his choices.

Wilbur's plan will also have a section on his general support needs. These may include any tasks he needs assistance or support in. This section will probably not contain a list of training objectives for Wilbur. Essential Lifestyle Planning has moved away from the notion that Wilbur will need to learn new skills in order to have the opportunity to have a life. Instead, we are really implementing a support model where Wilbur is already ready to have a life. All he needs is the proper support from us.

WHAT ABOUT GOALS AND TRAINING PROGRAMS?

Does this mean Wilbur won't be learning new skills? I don't think so. It just means that he will learn through participation, a type of teaching we will talk more about in Chapter 7. We will give him as much assistance as he needs—and no more. He will then be doing what he wants to do, in the way he wants to do it, and as independently as he is capable of.

But what if you are working in an ICF-MR style system? Will the kind of plan we're putting together with Wilbur meet the requirements for "active treatment" and goals that are "measurable and time limited?" I think it can. The intent of the "active treatment" requirement is that Wilbur not be sitting around all day doing nothing. And Wilbur and his Mom will certainly come up with goals that are measurable and time limited. They want to be sure we're accountable for doing what we said we would do, and they want it done by a particular time. We can do that.

I have used Essential Lifestyle Planning as an example of planning that is truly person centered. There are other models that also accomplish the same goal. If you want to know more about these models or if you'd like training in a specific model, refer to the Resources section for websites and contact information.

To review, truly person-centered planning:
- Asks the right questions (or makes good observations)
- Of the right people (the person whose plan it is and his circle of friends)
- To support personal choice,
- Personal routines,
- Informal training,
- And real outcomes

SELF-DETERMINATION—
THE REVOLUTION OF RISING EXPECTATIONS

Person-centered planning, in some form or other, has been around for a number of years. As long as I have been in this business, we have been telling people "it's your life" or "you're the boss" or "you have rights." Most of this has been lip service. We said the person was in charge, but we went ahead and made the decisions anyway. If someone piped up and told us plainly what he wanted, we would usually put on our long professional faces and judge whether or not the request was "appropriate." "Appropriate" usually meant something we professionals would like or find acceptable. Sometimes "appropriate" just meant "available." If someone asked for something we couldn't provide, we labeled their request "inappropriate."

Over the years a strange thing happened. Many of the people we supported took us seriously. They began to ask why. They began to ask why not. One young man, frustrated by the interdisciplinary team's inability to listen to his needs, said, "Well, why don't you just give me the money you spend on me and let me take care of my own needs!" What that young man was talking about is now known as "self-determination."

Self-determination has created what left-wing political thinkers used to call "a revolution of rising expectations." If you lead someone to expect something better, you'd better be prepared to deliver. Or he'll run over you in his attempt to get what he wants. As Bob Dylan said to the "mothers and fathers throughout the land…" "your old road is rapidly agin' /Please get out of the new one if you can't lend a hand/'Cause the times they are a changin'." Getting out of the road and lending a hand to people with disabilities so they can run their own lives is self-determination.

CONTROL OVER RESOURCES

Michael Smull says the two ingredients of self-determination are "planning for your future and control over resources." You can make plans all day long, but they will be glittering pie in the sky if there is no way they can be achieved. Self-determination, at its core, means control over resources.

An enormous amount of money is spent every year on supports for people with disabilities. This money is most often controlled by legislatures, regulatory agencies and case managers (who decide who gets what from the services that are available). The usual way for the money to be allocated is through what is called "categorical funding." What that means is that different "categories" of disability or types of support get different kinds of funding amounts. The different types of funding are usually called "slots." When a slot becomes open, a person is "placed" into it. Sounds pretty confining, eh? Is this the way you would like to live?

Let's see how categorical funding might work for Deborah. Since Deborah has moderate mental retardation and cerebral palsy, she can probably get money for "developmental disability services." These services may include "skill training," "vocational training," and "residential support." Each person in Deborah's category is entitled to a certain amount of money for each category of service. Skill training will probably be offered in the form of classes in the sheltered workshop or a personal trainer who will teach Deborah how to do tasks more independently. Vocational training will likely be some kind of made up "prevocational" classes that are supposed to get Deborah "ready" for a real job. And "residential support" could be the choice between institutional or group home placement, and "supported living" with constant staff presence (see Chapter 13, "A Home and a Job in the Real World" for more on residential and vocational options).

Most of these services are provided by agencies that specialize in a particular kind of program. These agencies may have open "slots" that they or Deborah's case manager offer to Deborah. The sheltered workshop may have a place at a table bagging screws. The group home provider may have a "bed" in a home with other people with disabilities and round the clock staff. That's what they offer. That's what you get. Take it or leave it.

But what if one of Deborah's "must have's" is to continue to live with her parents, but they need training and financial support to make that possible? What if she doesn't want a "trainer" who will teach her new skills, but just a "companion" who will spend time with her, giving whatever support she needs, as she goes about her life (experiencing informal learning)? What if she wants to learn a job the way everyone else does—on the job? Unless Deborah has control over the way money is spent on her, she will not be able to pursue any of these creative options. She will only get the services that are provided in open slots.

And what if Deborah changes her mind about what she wants? Will the system be responsive to her changes, or will it hold her back, saying she isn't "ready" for something new and exciting?

Sadly, Deborah and her family will probably give up trying to change the system. They will take what's offered. It usually seems better than nothing.

Control of resources starts with person-centered planning. Instead of a case manager or interdisciplinary team doing an assessment and determining what Deborah needs, those needs will be decided by Deborah herself (with the help of family, friends, and advocates).

Instead of a slot that Deborah can be placed into, she will have an authorized budget amount. The money would be allocated to Deborah, not to a program or agency or disability. That amount of money (reviewed and changed at least annually) can be spent in various ways to support the desires Deborah has expressed. Deborah might have a personal advocate or "support broker" who will help her choose services, stay within the budgeted amount, and make adjustments as necessary. She might even have a "business agent" who will help hire and pay providers Deborah decides to contract with. Deborah's agent could also provide an accounting system to show how the money is being spent and assist in cost-findings that will be part of the next year's budget process.

PARTICIPANT DRIVEN SERVICES

This kind of system, where the person who uses the services is in charge of how the money is spent is sometimes called "participant driven services." This is way outside the box thinking in some places. It requires a change in the way everyone does business.

We have already seen that the first change is for the planning process to truly be person centered.

Next, decisions about resources (money) have to be put in the hands of the people who use the services. If this is going to be meaningful, the public mental health system can't be the only game in town. It's not meaningful choice if, as they used to say about the Model T Ford, "you can have any color you want, as long as it's black."

There also have to be enough service providers to choose from. With the people who receive support services in charge of how the money is spent, there would be a lot of competition for their business. There might be provider fairs where all of those agencies that operate group homes or workshops or supported living or supported employment programs (or something else for which a market demand arises) can strut their stuff. The person with the budget (and his friends, advocates, brokers, etc.) can then shop around for the nicest people, the best deal, and the type of support that most meets his needs. Wouldn't you want to work in that kind of environment? You would be sure that the person you support chose you to do the work. You would have to meet his needs, or he could fire you. I've been a service provider, and I'd rather sell my services directly to the person who uses them than to a government agency.

We will have to be careful, though, that we don't turn self-determination into just another piece of the system. If I sell "self-determination services" to a person with disabilities, I'll probably still be the one in charge.

We professionals must constantly take a back seat and know our place if people with disabilities are truly to be in charge of their own lives. We will have to bite our tongues when we start judging a person's dreams as "appropriate" or not. We will have to fasten our seat belts and prepare for the bumpy ride that is life lived by real people in the real world.

Self-determination is a way of thinking whose time has come. It will come sooner in some areas than in others. You can be part of the change. There are exciting times ahead.

SELF-ADVOCACY

I like to travel around to different conferences and training sessions to see what people are doing. Not long ago I was privileged to spend a day in a session on Common Vision led by the people from ACT (Advocating Change Together). ACT was founded in 1979 in Minneapolis, MN "in response to the growing concern that individuals with developmental disabilities were being isolated and excluded from decisions regarding their lives" (to quote their literature). It is an organization operated by and for people with disabilities.

At the session I attended, we had group singing and a slide show about the history of how people with disabilities have been viewed and treated. But for me the high point of the day was a private conversation I had with a woman during one of the breaks. Gloria Steinbring travels with the ACT group to tell her story. It is a story of institutionalization and abuse. But it is also a story of hope. Gloria has found her voice through ACT, and it's a voice that annoys and disturbs many in the corridors of power.

Gloria told me about one issue that is particularly close to her. At the state-run facility where she and her husband lived for many years there is a graveyard. The graves are marked by rows of short concrete blocks with numbers on them. They are the graves of all the anonymous people, including Gloria's husband, who died in that place. Gloria and her friends at ACT did not want those people to be forgotten. So they asked the State of Minnesota for the records that showed the names that went with the numbers on the markers. The state said that was "confidential" information and refused to turn it over. ACT members demonstrated at the state capitol. Then they sued the state—and won. They have the names that go with the stones. It turns out there are 10,000 such stones across the state. Now ACT and others are raising money to pay for putting names on all of the markers. Gloria is proud of her work. She is proud of herself. She has become a self-advocate.

Self-advocates are everywhere. They are speaking up and speaking out. They are rocking the boat and demanding that people think outside the box. You can support the process.

You can encourage the people you support to become familiar with political issues (like categorical funding or anonymous gravestones). You can help families clarify what they truly want and make them aware of what options are available. You can help people form self-advocacy groups that get people talking together about common concerns.

Self-advocacy is a way of exercising the most important right we have in a free country—the right to be heard, the right to stand up (or raise your fist) and be counted. (For more on exercising rights, see Chapter 10, "A Matter of Rights.")

LITTLE BY LITTLE

Little steps are important, not only because each step brings progress; but also because even small progress encourages people to try for more.

Advocacy means not always being nice. Nothing will change if we are not willing to rattle a few cages and threaten the status quo. But we also have to remember that it has taken many small victories to get this far, and we've still got a long way to go. Little steps are important, not only because each step brings progress; but also because even small progress encourages people to try for more. Don't get discouraged by the frustrating pace of change. Never think you are not making a difference.

The story is told of a man walking on a beach as the tide is running out. Far in the distance, he sees another person walking along the water's edge. Every few seconds the person approaching reaches down and then throws something into the water. As the man gets closer, he sees that this other person on the beach is a woman, and he sees that what she is throwing are starfish.

Puzzled by her strange behavior, the man asks the woman, "Why are you throwing those starfish into the surf?"

The woman smiles and replies, "Because the tide is going out, and the ones left stranded on the shore will dry out and die."

The man is amused by the futility of her efforts. He says condescendingly, "But Madam, there are millions of starfish on this beach. Throwing a few into the surf can't possibly make a difference."

The woman just smiles, tosses another starfish to freedom and says, "Made a difference to that one."

Chapter 5

"MENTAL RETARDATION" RECONSIDERED

I confessed in the first chapter that when I started to work at Colin Anderson Center I didn't really know what "mental retardation" was. I thought I would learn from working with the people who lived there. But the people were all so different from each other that I still couldn't figure out was the common thread, the reason everyone said they had mental retardation. Some of the people I met looked very different from anyone else I'd ever seen. Others looked like anyone I might meet on the street; but when I tried to talk with them, they just stared at me or made sounds I couldn't understand. Then there were those who didn't talk at all but who seemed to know what was going on. Some of them seemed very smart to me, in their own way.

Over the years, I've met hundreds of people who are said to have developmental disabilities and mental retardation. I've learned enough about the official definitions to be able to be a contributing member of various planning teams. I've helped with IQ tests and can usually estimate which of the four ranges of mental retardation a person will fall into.

But I'm still not sure I know what mental retardation *is*. Fortunately, I'm not alone. The American Association on Mental Retardation (AAMR) currently has a working group that is trying to come up with a new definition that will make use of what we've learned since the last definition was written in the early 1990's. As you can imagine, the discussions are sometimes intense.

You need to know what most people are talking about when they use some key words, but I'd also like you to be sensitive to some of the issues that are involved when we try to define something as broad and variable as mental retardation.

"DISABILITIES"—DIFFERENT FROM NORMAL

I use the word "disabilities" a lot. That's because the focus of this book, and of my work, is people who are considered to have disabilities. But what is a disability, anyway?

Some advocacy groups have tried to get rid of the word "disability" altogether, suggesting alternatives like "differently abled." But the fact is that the word disability is firmly rooted in the world of human services (as witness the recent Americans with Disabilities Act—ADA). You will be dealing with service and advocacy agencies, funding sources and clinical disciplines that all specialize in supports for people with particular types of disability. We need to use the word "disability" in a way that honors and respects the value of the people it is applied to.

When I'm looking for definitions, I always start with the dictionary. While it won't tell us everything we need to know, it will give us a place to start.

My fat Webster's unabridged dictionary defines "disability" as something that makes a person "unable or unfit" or which "deprives of normal strength or power." I don't particularly like the way that sounds, especially the part about "unable or unfit."

And what does "normal" mean? What would "normal strength or power" look like? "Normal" is what is usual, average, standard, or expected. Most people can walk without assistance. Walking is considered "normal." So a person who cannot walk functions differently from the normal, or expected, way. She is considered to have a "disability" with regard to walking.

I slipped in another word there that needs a definition of its own. The word is "function." I said the woman who cannot work "functions" differently. The way something functions is the way it works or operates. We even say that the purpose of something is its function, as in, "The function of legs is getting from place to place." If legs don't do their job as intended, they are not functioning in the normal way.

57

When we talk about the normal functioning of a human body and mind, we are talking about the parts of the body doing what they seem to be designed to do. Hands usually grasp objects; tongues and mouths usually form words; brains usually learn from experience and solve problems. Those activities are the usual functions of hands and tongues and brains. A person with a disability is a person whose body and mind don't function in the usual ways.

Something about the person with a disability works in a different way than with most people. That doesn't mean that the people who have what we call disabilities are "deficient" or "defective." It doesn't mean that they can't have rich, full, satisfying lives. It just means that they will do life's activities in different ways, because their tools function differently from what is "normal."

Be careful, here. Thinking of a disability as some level of functioning that is not "normal" gets us into some tricky territory. For example, being 7'4" tall is certainly not "normal," but if it means you can easily put a round ball through a high hoop, it wouldn't be considered a "disability." If the person used his "abnormal" height to play good basketball, we'd consider it a gift. Why are some ways of not being normal not considered to be disabilities?

It gets even trickier. What about the man who was born deaf who refused to allow his daughter, who was also deaf, to have a cochlear implant that would let her hear? He argued passionately that not being able to hear is not a "disability." He said agreeing with the doctors that his daughter had something "wrong" with her that needed to be "fixed" meant that he also felt there was something wrong with him, that he wasn't an acceptable human being. What do you think?

DEVELOPMENTAL DISABILITIES

Now that we know what disabilities are, it should be easy to figure out what "developmental" disabilities are. They are disabilities that delay or change a person's development and growth.

Human beings are not formed instantly. We develop from single cells into embryos, then into babies, then into children, then into adults. Most of our development happens from conception until adulthood (usually considered to be age 18). We call that period of time the "developmental period."

During the developmental period, each of our body's functions develops according to a complicated set of instructions. The instructions, contained in our DNA, tell the body's building blocks how to construct brains and legs and eyes and all the other marvelous organs that help us live in the world.

This building process never unfolds in exactly the same way. That's why we're so different from each other. Sometimes eyes come out blue, sometimes brown. Some eyes see things clearly at a distance; others don't see anything at all. When the instructions cause some part of a person's body to be built in a way that it doesn't work (function) the way that part usually works, we say the person has a "developmental disability."

In addition to good genetic instructions, normal development requires a healthy environment. Give the developing body drugs instead of food, or abuse instead of love, and things won't come out the way they're supposed to.

A developmental disability, then, is a change in a person's functioning that occurs sometime during the developmental period and delays or changes normal development.

In the charts below, I have listed some of the most common developmental disabilities, as well as some of the things that cause developmental disabilities to happen.

SOME DEVELOPMENTAL DISABILITIES:

Mental Retardation
People with mental retardation are those who develop at a below average rate and experience difficulty in learning and social adjustment.

Cerebral Palsy
Cerebral palsy is a term used to describe a group of chronic conditions affecting body movement and muscle coordination. It is caused by damage to one or more specific areas of the brain, usually occurring during fetal development; before, during, or shortly after birth; or during infancy. "Cerebral" refers to the brain and "palsy" to muscle weakness/poor control.

Autism
Autism impacts the normal development of the brain in the areas of social interaction and communication skills (language). Children and adults with autism typically have difficulties in verbal and non-verbal communication, social interactions, and leisure or play activities. The disorder makes it hard for them to communicate with others and relate to the outside world. In some cases, aggressive and/or self-injurious behavior may be present.

Epilepsy (seizure disorder)
A brain disorder which causes repeated seizures, the form of which may range from a brief staring episode or sudden drop attack to a massive, prolonged, life-threatening convulsion. Seizures are often present in people who have mental retardation and cerebral palsy.

SOME CAUSES OF DEVELOPMENTAL DISABILITIES:

Pre-natal (before birth)
Rh incompatibility, poor nutrition, infections (Rubella, Syphilis, AIDS), radiation, drugs and alcohol, genetic defects (Down syndrome, fragile X), metabolic imbalances (PKU) NOTE: *Fetal Alcohol Syndrome (caused by the mother drinking alcohol during pregnancy) has become the leading known cause of mental retardation in western civilization. (Journal of American Medical Association, 1991) Each year in the US, 5,000 babies are born with Fetal Alcohol Syndrome (FAS). As many as 50,000 babies are born with an alcohol-related disability. (March of Dimes, 1992)*

Peri-natal (during birth)
Pre- or post-mature (being born too early or too late), presentation (the baby being born feet first or in another position that causes difficulty with delivery), anesthesia, multiple births, loss of oxygen

Post-natal (childhood)
Physical trauma (accident or child abuse), disease, drugs and chemicals, poor nutrition

HANDICAPS

If a disability means a person functions in a way that's different from "normal," what is a "handicap"? Going back to the dictionary, we find that the word "handicap" originally meant the extra weight put on fast racehorses to make the race fairer for the slower runners. From that meaning, handicap came to mean any burden placed upon some people that makes it harder to run the race. People with disabilities are "handicapped" because there are things in life that are harder for them to do because of the disability.

Let's consider a person who has the disability we call "paraplegia (pair-uh-PLEEDJ-uh)," a paralysis of the lower part of the body. One of his handicaps (one of the things he has difficulty doing) might be that he can't get to the upper bleacher seats at the ballgame.

Now think about this: Is it the fact that his legs don't move that causes the handicap? Or is it the fact that the bleacher seats are accessible only to people who can walk? You've probably guessed that I'm going to say it's the bleachers. And you're right. I say that it's barriers (like bleacher steps or heavy doors or closed minds) that cause handicaps. Why should life be unusually difficult just because some part of a person doesn't function in the usual way?

This idea, that it is obstacles, rather than disabilities, that cause handicaps, should give you great encouragement as a provider of supports. Why? Because unless you are a physician or medical researcher, you probably can't do anything about disabilities, the differences in functioning that many people are born with. You can't make paralyzed legs move or blind eyes see. You can't jump-start brains that are slow to figure things out. But you certainly can work to remove or overcome barriers and obstacles that keep people with differently functioning legs, eyes, and brains from participating fully in life in the real world.

We all have parts that don't function as well as they might. We try to accept ourselves as we are and do the best we can with what we have. But we must never accept handicaps, the obstacles put in the way of people who function in the ways that are called disabilities. Instead, it is our job to find ways over, under, around, or through the obstacles people encounter in their lives.

GIFTS AND GAPS

Nobody likes to be labeled. Labels make a person stand out for one particular characteristic, like "fat" or "dumb" or "shy." Labels keep us from getting to know the whole person.

"Disabled" and "handicapped" are labels that call attention to what is seen as wrong with a person. If we see "a disabled person," we're likely to lose sight of Tom or Ann. We see the things Tom and Ann can't do and miss the gifts they bring to our lives (Tom has a great sense of humor, and Ann is a hard worker).

I'd like to propose a way to get past labeling. I suggest that instead of putting people in different boxes labeled with what's "wrong" with them, we think of *all people* as having "gifts and gaps."

Our gifts are the things we're good at. I, for instance, am good with words. It is a gift I think I was born with, an inheritance from my magazine editor father. You, on the other hand, may have a gift for music, or athletics, or getting along well with other people.

Our gaps are the things we have trouble with. We all have them. I am terrible at math or anything else involving numbers. You might have trouble reading or speaking in public or learning new dance steps.

A disability is, from this perspective, a "gap," something a person needs help with. There's no shame in that. We've all got gaps in our abilities. We all need help with some things. None of us expects the things we're not good at to keep us from living full lives.

Envisioning all people as having both gifts and gaps means no one gets put into any labeled boxes. We're all human beings who are good at some things and need help with others. Everyone has both gifts and gaps. What are your gifts? What are your gaps?

We all try to use our gifts to have a successful and fulfilling life. We choose activities that take advantage of our giftedness. And we find ways to get around our gaps. We avoid situations that point out our lack of ability. Or we get help, develop support systems, and learn new skills.

My granddaughter Sarah seems to be gifted in seeing things visually and understanding diagrams, some of the areas I'm not so good at. And she has had difficulty reading, an area in which I excel. When we used to put together things like bicycles and bookcases, I would read the step-by-step instructions, and she would look at the pictures. Together we had a better understanding than either of us would have had separately. We overcame our gaps by taking advantage of each other's gifts.

This idea of gifts and gaps gets rid of labels because it includes everyone. No one is seen as so gifted that they don't need help and support sometimes. And no one is seen as having so many gaps in their skills that we don't need to recognize and take advantage of their gifts. Since everyone is gifted in some way, our job is to help people use their gifts to overcome their gaps.

MENTAL RETARDATION—DEFINITION

I said I don't like labels. But I also said our largest professional organization (AAMR) is working on a new definition. Why the contradiction?

There is a good reason for having a clear, descriptive definition of mental retardation, although we run the danger of labeling and stigmatizing people. That reason is that we as a society have decided that people who have this developmental disability are entitled by law to certain services and supports. The definition of mental retardation gives clear, measurable guidelines for who gets disability support services.

This question of definition, then, is important to the lives of a lot of people. There are approximately 7 million people in the United States who, using the current definition, have some degree of mental retardation. About 2 million of these people will need ongoing supports and assistance throughout their lives. Of these, 300,000 or so people are still on waiting lists to receive appropriate services.

I wish it were otherwise. I wish anyone who needed supports for a successful life could get them. A person wouldn't have to be labeled with a diagnosis in order to get needed treatment or support. But my wish is probably a long way off. In the meantime, you will need to understand the "official" definition of mental retardation so you understand how it is decided who gets support and who doesn't.

Most people in our field use the revised definition of mental retardation that was put forth by the AAMR (American Association on Mental Retardation) in 1992. This definition says there are three things that must be present in order for a person to be diagnosed as having mental retardation:

I. "Significantly sub-average intellectual functioning"

II. Occurs before age 18

III. Involves "related difficulties in two or more life skills areas," those areas being:

1. Communication—Does the person have difficulty making her wants and needs known? Can she express how she feels and what she prefers? Do other people understand her?

2. Self-care—Can the person dress and feed himself? Can he bathe, brush his teeth, comb his hair?

3. Home living—Does the person have difficulty preparing meals, paying her bills, cleaning house?

4. Social skills—Does he have difficulty relating to other people? Does he know how to make friends, date, attend social events?

5. Community use—Can she get to the store, register to vote, attend a public event?

6. Self-direction—Does he understand the consequences of his actions? Can he make long- and short-term plans and follow through with them?

7. Health and safety—Does she know what to do when she's sick? Would she walk into a busy street, go away with a stranger, recognize household dangers?

8. Functional academics—Can he read, write, and do simple arithmetic at a level sufficient to get along in the community?

9. Leisure—Can she occupy her free time safely and productively? Does she know how to engage in leisure time activities?

10. Work—Can he do a productive job in an integrated environment?

Let's start with the first item and work our way through the three parts of this definition.

INTELLECTUAL FUNCTIONING

The first part of the definition says that a person with mental retardation has "intellectual functioning" that is "significantly sub-average." In order for that to mean anything, we need to look at what "intelligence" is and what "average" means.

At first glance, intelligence is something we all understand. A person who is intelligent is someone we think of as "smart" or "bright," and one who is not very intelligent is thought of as "dumb" or "dull." You can probably give a rough estimate of whether you think one person is smarter than another. But *how* do you do that? What exactly are we comparing when we say one person is smarter than another? What is this thing we call "intelligence?"

Those are hard questions; and researchers are coming up with new ideas every day about intelligence and how the mind works. For our purposes here, I'd like to propose we think of "intelligence" as having to do with three things: quickness, depth, and flexibility.

First we look at how fast a person learns things. Does it take lots of repetition; or do they get it right away? We even refer to this characteristic in our everyday language. We say, "She's really quick" or "He's a little slow." It's important to realize that the word "retarded" means "slowed down or delayed." Many experts believe people with mental retardation develop in the same way as people without mental retardation, but at a slower rate. Others suggest that people with mental retardation have difficulties in particular areas of basic thinking and learning such as attention, perception, or memory

The next question that we ask in determining intelligence is "How deep does the person's knowledge go?" Sometimes a person seems intelligent at first glance, but you then find that their thinking is all on the surface. A person understands the simple outlines of things but doesn't seem to have the ability to go more deeply into them. When we refer to "rocket science," as in "It's not rocket science," we're talking about something that is complicated, with lots of connections between the individual bits of knowledge. We think of Einstein as being really intelligent because he was able to think deeply into things and understand how they are connected.

Finally, flexibility is one of the factors you get when you combine quickness and depth. A mind that quickly looks deeply into things can come up with new responses to situations it has never been in before. People with flexible minds are able to solve problems, create new solutions and think outside the box. An inflexible mind, on the other hand, tends to follow deep grooves of thinking that have been developed laboriously over time.

Howard has mental retardation. He seems to show just the opposite of these characteristics of intelligence. He is slow to learn. It is frustrating for his parents and friends that Howard just doesn't "get it." "How many times do I have to tell you?" says Mom in frustration. The answer to that question may be "many, many, many." That is why patience is so important when working with people who have mental retardation. Howard may have to be told and shown and guided over and over before he learns how to do the things that get him what he wants. And, once he has figured out how something works, Howard may want things to stay reliable and consistent. He doesn't want to have to learn a whole new way of doing things.

People with quick minds usually like newness. They thrive on situations that always change. Such situations keep their minds active, keep them from getting bored. Lily's mind works more slowly, and she is threatened by that same novelty. Lily prefers a secure routine that she knows she can follow. She is successful in the things she knows how to do. It took Lily two months to finally learn how to put her clothes away so they wouldn't get wrinkled and she'd be able to find them when she wants to. You're really going to mess her up if you decide to change the system.

And finally, many people who have mental retardation have a simple and unsophisticated understanding of things, an understanding that may work alright for simple matters but which doesn't go very deep. Our challenge is to realize that such simplicity can be a "gift," not a "gap." It doesn't take a lot of what we call "intelligence" to have simple common sense. Sometimes I wonder if a high level of intelligence is not a curse of complexity. Those of us with high IQ's spin our minds in worrisome circles trying to figure everything out. My mother used to say, "For somebody who's supposed to be so smart, you sure do a lot of dumb things."

MEASURING INTELLIGENCE

An IQ (Intelligence Quotient) score is supposed to be a number which tells how smart you are. A psychologist administers the IQ test by asking the subject (we'll call her Suzy) to answer questions and solve problems. The test items are arranged in the order in which people usually develop new thinking abilities as they grow up. Easy questions first; hard questions as the test goes on. The early items on the test are things a small child should be able to figure out.

Take for example this simple task, known as an "analogy"—"Trees are green; butter is _____." You immediately fill in the word "yellow." The answer didn't seem to take much thinking; but if you look carefully at it, you'll realize your mind quickly did a number of things. When you heard "Trees are green," you knew the sentence was indicating the color (green) of the subject (trees). Then when you heard "butter is..." you knew that the tester wanted you to fill in the *color* of butter. You also happen to *know* the color of butter. So you answered the question easily. A normal five-year old might have to think about the question a little more, but he could still get the answer. Not so for some people who have mental retardation. I have heard adults, after thinking hard about the problem, give answers like "I don't know," "I forgot," or "...good on toast." It's not that they don't know what butter and trees are. It's that they don't understand quickly what the question is. Their brains don't figure out the analogy.

Back to our IQ test. The tester keeps asking Suzy to answer the items until she is "stumped" and can answer no more. The test items are in order of difficulty (the order in which developing humans usually learn things), so an age level can be assigned to each test item.

Let's say the last items Suzy got right are those that are usually answered correctly by a five-year-old. This gives the tester Suzy's "mental age"—five years. "Mental age" is another of those slippery ideas that gets us in trouble if we're not careful. Suzy's mental age of five years means that she can work out the kinds of thinking problems a typical five-year-old can work out. It does not mean she "has the mind of a five-year-old" because it happens that Suzy is 45 years old (her "chronological age"). She has had a lot of life experiences the average five-year-old knows nothing about. But the test does indicate that there is a significant (serious, important) gap between Suzy's tested ability to do thinking problems and the ability you would usually expect to see in a person her age.

How do we measure the gap? We use a formula that compares Suzy's chronological age (how long she's been on the planet) with her mental

67

age (the developmental level she achieves on the IQ test). The number we get is called IQ or "intelligence quotient." The higher the number, the more intelligent the person is said to be. IQ isn't supposed to measure what you know or what you learned in school. It, rather, tells us how well your mind works, assigns that a number, and compares it with others who take the same test.

The notion that IQ can be measured in this way is very controversial. Some people say the tests are tilted in favor of the things that college-educated, white males (the people who made up most of the tests) think makes people smart. These people say the tests are "culturally biased." That means that some groups may score lower on the tests because of the way they were raised or the way they see the world.

Others say there are different kinds of intelligence, like "emotional intelligence" or "spatial intelligence," and that the tests only measure "cognitive" (problem-solving, reasoning) intelligence.

Still others put forth the idea that intelligence seems to be inherited and is therefore affected by who your parents are.

For our purposes now, we just have to know that intelligence, as measured by IQ tests, is one of the determining factors in a diagnosis of mental retardation.

The definition of mental retardation says it involves intelligence that is "significantly" below average. What does that mean?

If we're going to know who's average and who's below average, we'll have to have some numbers to go on. The following graph shows the distribution of IQ scores in an average population.

Chapter 5 – "Mental Retardation" Reconsidered

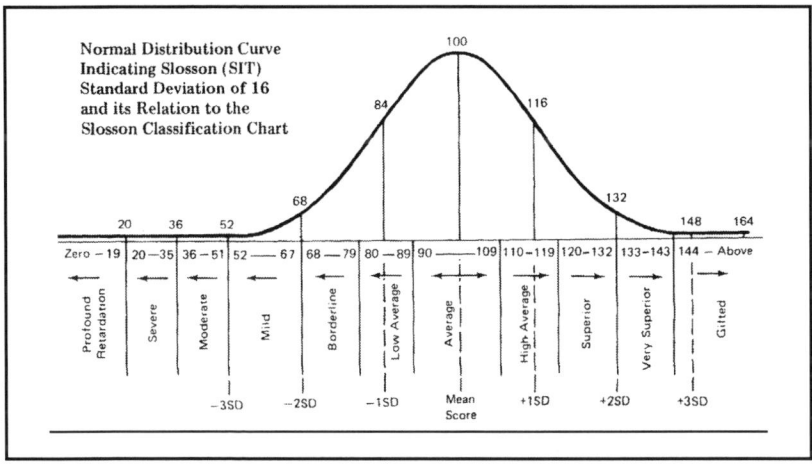

The shape of the graph is known as a "bell curve" (because if you use your imagination you can see the shape of a bell, with its clapper hanging down around the 100 line). The horizontal line at the bottom of the graph represents IQ scores, from lower to higher. The height of the vertical lines represents how many people in a normal sample would have each test score.

A score of 100 is considered average; and, not surprisingly, we see that most people's scores fall right around 100. As we move to the right on the graph, to higher scores, we see that fewer and fewer people have the higher scores, until the number of people considered to be in the "Gifted" range (above 148) is very small indeed.

Going the other way, we find a lot of people in the "Low Average" and "Borderline" areas, but once we get below an IQ of 68, we have "significantly" fewer people. An IQ below 68 is considered (on this test, the Slosson) to be "significantly sub-average intellectual functioning." That score puts the person in the area considered to be mental retardation.

Below the cut-off for mental retardation, you see four more groups. These are the "ranges" of mental retardation—Mild, Moderate, Severe and Profound. These are not really precise indicators, and they are not used by many clinicians. They just give a shorthand way of talking about a person's general level of intellectual functioning. Special Educators tend to refer to people in the Mild range as "Educable," those in the Moderate range as "Trainable," and those in the lowest ranges as "Severe and Profound."

69

Even better than putting people with mental retardation into categories of "functioning level" is to consider how much support they need in order to overcome the handicaps presented by their disabilities. The AAMR now uses four support levels:

Intermittent Support—support on an "as needed basis." Support that is not needed on a continuous daily basis.

Limited Support—support over a limited time span, such as transition from school to work or to job training.

Extensive Support—support needed on a daily basis, but not necessarily in all life areas.

Pervasive Support—constant support that may include life-sustaining measures. Daily support across all life areas.

Notice that these categories of support are concerned less with what is "wrong" with the person and more with what we, as support providers, need to do. That's a good step in the direction of helping people use their gifts to compensate for their gaps.

A "DEVELOPMENTAL" DISABILITY

The second part of the definition of mental retardation says that it "occurs before age 18." As we said above, this age of onset makes mental retardation a "developmental" disability; that is, whatever caused the condition happened during the age of development (before adulthood).

A person who has already reached adulthood could end up with "significantly sub-average intellectual functioning" from having injured his head in an accident, but this would not be called "mental retardation." Though that person might get a low score on an IQ test and need help with many daily tasks, the condition would be referred to as Traumatic Brain Injury (TBI) or Acquired Brain Injury (ABI). As you will see, such a distinction makes little difference in the way you support a person. The distinction is made only because funding and support services available for the two groups of people are very different.

Remember that the "retardation" part of mental retardation refers to a slowing down. And what is slowed down by this disability is a person's development; that is, learning the skills and abilities that usually come with growing up.

LIFE SKILLS DIFFICULTIES

The third part of the definition is "related difficulties in 2 or more" of the life skills areas listed above. These difficulties are the things a person has trouble doing because of his mental retardation. This is what I earlier called a "handicap." You will also remember that I said that while the disability (whatever brain dysfunction causes the lower IQ) cannot be "healed," the handicap (the things the person has difficulty doing because of the disability) can be overcome.

The life skills on the list are often referred to as "adaptive skills," because they help a person adapt, or adjust, to various life circumstances. There are many checklists that measure the extent of a person's adaptive skills. We used to use these checklists to tell us what skills the person would have to be trained in. Now we are more likely to use these checklists to tell us what kinds of supports the person will need.

Here's an interesting question: If, because of the great training and support you provide, the person with mental retardation is now able to participate fully in all of the life skills areas on the list, would she still have mental retardation? The IQ test score has not changed; the only thing that is different is the person's life skills. It's a controversial question, the answer to which revolves around a word we've already encountered—independence. Some people would say that if the person cannot participate in all life areas *independently*, she still has "related difficulties" in those areas. Others would say that we all have "difficulties" (gaps) with some of the areas, and we shouldn't set a higher standard of independence than we set for ourselves. What do you think?

Another question about this imaginary person who has met parts 1 and 2 of the definition of mental retardation, but who has managed to overcome the life skills difficulties through supports and opportunities is, Would it be a good thing to consider him "cured" and remove the label of mental retardation from his life? Think carefully. What if some of the supports he still needs are paid for by services that are only available to people with disabilities? If he no longer had mental retardation, he would lose some of the (publicly funded) supports that caused him to lose the label. This is a tricky issue, and it points up the necessity of helping someone develop "natural supports" in her life—family, friends, neighbors and co-workers who can offer her the supports and assistance she needs, so she does not have to rely on the disability system. Natural supports cannot be taken away by a change in definition or a new test score.

The definition of "mental retardation" is something that will change over time as intelligent, caring people set their minds to the issues of how best to support people who are different from normal but who should be fully included in all of life's possibilities.

Chapter 6

THE ABC'S OF LEARNING

HABILITATION—
TRAINING, TRAINING, TRAINING

When the ICF-MR regulations came to Colin Anderson Center, training was something new to us. We had never had the time (or the inclination) to teach people new skills. Our job had just been to take care of them. I've already mentioned one of the "radical" requirements of the new regulations—everyone had to have a plan. Well, the plan led to goals, and the goals led to training. From the time people got up in the morning (dressing, bedmaking, toothbrushing) to the time they went to bed at night (undressing, bathing, toothbrushing), people had training programs. We ran training programs for self-feeding, for toileting, for putting on shoes and pants and bras, for attending to task and following simple commands and using manual sign language.

All of this training was being done because the ICF-MR regulations required us to provide "active treatment" during almost every waking hour. The active treatment requirement was to eliminate all the sitting around that was the usual activity on the old wards. But "active treatment" came to mean "training", because the ICF-MR regulations were a "Habilitation Model" of services.

The word "habilitation" comes from the Latin word *habilitare*, which means "to enable." The idea was that people were in institutions because they didn't know how to do things. If we taught them new skills, it would "enable" them to leave the institution and get a life.

73

BEHAVIORISM HAPPENS

In Chapter 2, we took a brief look at some of the educational theories popular at different times. I left out one of the most important theories for disability support services, because it more properly belongs in this chapter. I am referring to the theory of "behaviorism."

Proposed by John Watson in the early part of the twentieth century and extended by B.F. Skinner in the 1950's and 60's, behavioral psychology was concerned with why living things act the way they do. Animal studies suggested that all behavior was a response to a "stimulus," something that starts a chain of events that ends in some kind of action. Skinner, as the leader of the "radical behaviorists," believed there was nothing happening inside human beings but stimulus and response. What we commonly refer to as emotion and conscience and reason were all just stimulus and response learned through experience.

The first psychologists I met at Colin Anderson Center were behaviorists. They believed the behavior of people with mental retardation could be *shaped* by applying carefully researched techniques learned in training animals. These psychologists thought it didn't matter whether the people with developmental disabilities could "understand" what they were doing. They said a person's behavior, that is, what the person *does, is* the person. Change the behavior and you change the person.

Remember the part of the definition of mental retardation about "related difficulties in two or more life skills areas?" Those life skills areas are, according to behaviorists, simply behaviors. Using behavioral shaping techniques was seen as the way of teaching people new life skills that would overcome their "related difficulties." If a person could learn enough new life skills, he could be cured of mental retardation.

But how does this "shaping" and "learning" take place? That's what the behaviorists were studying.

Behavioral researchers studied animals to see how they learn to do new things. By observing closely, they broke the learning process down into three basic steps:

1. something happens before
2. animal does something
3. something happens after

They called these steps Antecedent (something that happens before), Behavior (something the animal does) and Consequence (something that happens after). A-B-C. Antecedent-Behavior-Consequence. Those three things and the way they relate to each other are the key to understanding the behavioral approach. It's probably as clear as mud right now, but bear with me. It'll all be straight in a minute.

BEHAVIOR—WHAT YOU DO

Let's start with B for Behavior. Behavior is, simply, *something you do*. It is an action. Other people can see you do it. That makes behavior different from feelings or thoughts (some behaviorists think feelings and thoughts are behaviors, too; but that's a longer story). When I see you do something, I don't know why you're doing it or what you think about it. I just see what you do. That's your Behavior.

According to the behaviorists, behavior doesn't "just happen." People (and rats and pigeons) do things because they've *learned* to act that way in particular circumstances. What I mean by "particular circumstances" is what happens just before the behavior (Antecedent) and what happens just after the behavior (Consequence).

ANTECEDENT—WHAT COMES BEFORE

The word "antecedent" comes from the Latin root *ante*, which means "before." If you're a poker player, you know that to "ante up" means to put money in the pot *before* you start to bet. If you are interested in historic homes, you know that an "antebellum" mansion is one that was built "before" (*ante*) the Civil War (*bellum*). An Antecedent comes *before* a Behavior *and causes it to happen*. The Antecedent is the stimulus. The Behavior is the response.

How did you wake up this morning? Perhaps the alarm clock made a loud noise. The alarm clock's noise *caused* you to wake up. The noise was the Antecedent, and waking up was the Behavior.

There are lots of these Antecedents in our daily lives. Sometimes they're called "cues." Cues lead you to do particular behaviors. An empty feeling in your stomach is a cue (Antecedent) to go to the kitchen and hunt for some breakfast (Behavior). A particular kind of music is the cue that your local weather forecast is coming on the TV. You turn your attention to the screen and turn up the volume (Behavior). A car horn honks (cue) in your driveway. You grab your jacket and lunchbox and head for the door (Behavior).

Another kind of Antecedent that is common in our lives is called a "prompt." A prompt is a way for one person to communicate to another what they would like the other to do (Behavior). A prompt may be a simple request, such as "Please come here." The request (prompt), when done nicely, causes you to come to me (Behavior). This kind of prompt is called "verbal," because it uses words. Verbal prompts are quite common in our world (though if they're too common, we call it nagging).

You don't need words for a prompt. Sometimes a prompt can be a gesture, like when your mother pointed at the spilled milk and extended a sponge toward you. Her gesture is a prompt that causes some cleaning up behavior on your part. If a person you're working with doesn't have good language (verbal) abilities, you may be able to communicate with her through gestures. And she may use gestures(pointing, directing her eyes, grabbing) to show you what she wants from you.

Sometimes Behavior needs a real kick in the pants to get going. We call this "physical assistance." When the dance instructor moves your arms and legs, his action physically assists you to do whatever Behavior he wants you to do. Physical assistance can also be used to move the hands of a person who, because of a cognitive disability, doesn't understand what you want him to do.

Cues and prompts (verbal, gestural, physical) are all antecedents that cause a behavior to happen. Once you understand this, you'll be aware of all of the antecedents in your environment.

CONSEQUENCE—WHAT COMES AFTER

OK; we've got A for Antecedent (what comes before) and B for Behavior (what you do). Finally we get to C, which stands for Consequence. A Consequence is something that *follows* (comes after) a behavior and *is caused by it*. That last part is important. In order for an event to be considered a *Consequence* of a particular behavior, the behavior has to *cause* the consequence to happen.

Let's say I'm trying to develop my reputation as a rainmaker. I invite a bunch of people to a grassy area in the park and lead them in a ritual dance that involves waving cans of baked beans over our heads. About an hour into the ritual, we wish the baked beans were umbrellas, because it has started to pour down rain. The rain *followed* (came after) the ritual dance. But did the dance *cause* it to rain? I'd like you to think so. But you understand that there's no relationship between my baked bean dance and the thunderstorm. You know that the rain was just a *coincidence*, not a *consequence* of our behavior. An event is a *consequence* of a behavior only if the behavior *causes* the event to occur.

Behavioral psychologists tell us there are basically two kinds of Consequence. (Ok, Mr. Behaviorist, I know that's an oversimplification. Remember; this is a "Beginner's Guide.") The two kinds of Consequence are called "reinforcer" and "punisher."

REINFORCERS AND PUNISHERS— TWO TYPES OF CONSEQUENCE

Let's take reinforcer first. The simple definition of a reinforcer has two parts. A reinforcer is:

- something you like and will work for, and
- if a reinforcer follows a behavior, the behavior is *more likely* to happen again.

That makes sense, doesn't it? If my action (Behavior) causes something good to happen to me, I'm going to want to do that behavior again. I want to get more reinforcers. They are things that I like and will work for.

Reinforcers are the heart of the behaviorist theory of learning. In order to teach any behavior, all you need to do is be sure that every time the person (pigeon, rat, dog) does the behavior you want, you immediately give them something they like. They will learn to do the behavior, in order to get the reinforcer. Another way of saying this is, "People do what they do to get what they want."

Before we go into more about how reinforcers work, let's get the (simplified) definition of a punisher. Remember that a punisher is another kind of Consequence—it comes after a Behavior, and is caused by it. A punisher, though, is just the *opposite* of a reinforcer. Can you work out the definition?

A punisher is:
- something you *don't* like and will try to avoid, and
- if a punisher follows a behavior, the behavior is *less likely* to happen again.

If every time you say the word "stupid" (Behavior) a little hand comes out of the sky and bops you on the nose (Consequence), don't you think you'd learn to change your language?

Reinforcers work to *increase* desired behaviors; and punishers work (in theory) to *decrease* unwanted behaviors. We'll deal with this a lot more in Chapter 9, "Why Does She Act That Way?"

A MOTIVATED PIGEON

Let's take a look at how the psychological researchers figured this stuff out.

Imagine you're back in Skinner's laboratory at Harvard. The walls are lined, floor to ceiling, with cages of pigeons. There is one pigeon to a cage. Why pigeons? Well, pigeons aren't the brightest lights. Their brains are about the size of the end of your little finger. Their behavior is pretty simple. So they should be easy to study.

Let's see if we can get the pigeon to do a new behavior; that is, whether we can "teach" it something.

We'll install a little lever on the side of the cage, placed so the pigeon can operate it by pecking it. And we'll set up the mechanism so that whenever the pigeon presses the lever, a pellet of tasty Purina Pigeon Chow drops into a little dish at the pigeon's feet. Press the lever, get the pellet. Simple.

You have set up the cage so the pigeon can get something it likes, but you can't explain stuff to pigeons. You can't just say "Hey, Pidge, press the lever and you get a tasty treat." They don't understand English (or French, for that matter). This is an experiment, anyway. We're trying to see whether a pigeon's behavior can be changed just by giving it a reward every time it does the desired behavior (pecking the lever). This isn't teaching in the sense of lecturing. Rather, it is *shaping behavior* by the use of reinforcers.

Chapter 6 – The ABC's of Learning

How are we going to tell if the experiment is working? Remember our definition of a reinforcer: it is something the pigeon likes and will work for (tasty Pigeon Chow) *and* if it follows a behavior (pecking the lever), the behavior is *more likely* to happen again. Looks like we're going to have to count behaviors (lever pecks) to see if they increase. This counting is called "data collection."

In order to collect data on the pigeon pressing the lever, we hook the lever to an automatic counting device. The device has a piece of paper in it that turns with a clock. Every time the pigeon presses the lever, a little pen makes a mark on the paper.

There's one more thing we have to do before we can run our experiment. In order to know whether our Pigeon Chow reward is working as a reinforcer (increasing the behavior), we have to know how many times the pigeon would peck the lever if he didn't get a reward. We call this number the *baseline*—the number we start out with before we do our experiment. So we turn on the machine that counts lever pecks (but not the one that delivers Pigeon Chow pellets) and put the pigeon in the cage.

We make sure the pigeon is hungry. That way he'll be really motivated to get that Pigeon Chow. But since the pigeon doesn't understand the device, he doesn't go straight for the reward. He just pecks around the cage aimlessly, trying to find something to eat. Sometimes he pecks the lever, but when he finds he can't eat it, he goes on to other things. Our data recording device keeps track of the lever pecks. It says in the first hour the pigeon pecked at the lever six times. We'll call that our *baseline rate*—six pecks per hour.

Now the fun begins. Remember, our theory is that if the pigeon is rewarded for pecking the lever, he'll learn that he can get food that way...and peck more often. Our baseline rate of six pecks an hour has told us how many times the pigeon will press the lever without a reward. In order to begin our experiment, we change the *conditions* of the cage. In research a "condition" is the environment the research subject is in. A condition that is changed to test its impact on the subject is called a "variable." Our new condition is that when the pigeon pecks the lever he gets "something he likes and will work for." What should happen to the rate of lever pecks? Right; they should increase. Let's watch.

The pigeon is put into the cage and does his usual pecking around. He hits the lever and hears the clink of the chow pellet in the dish. He immediately recognizes it as one of his favorites and gobbles it up. What does he do next? Well, if you think pigeons are really smart, you might say he'll peck the lever again to get another pellet. But the fact is his little pigeon brain hasn't gotten the connection between the lever and the food. So he goes back to pecking around. He hits the lever again, and again he gets the food. At the end of the first hour, we check the data recording device and find that the pigeon has pecked the lever 10 times. That's a little higher than our baseline but still not enough of an increase to prove anything. We continue the experiment. At the end of the second hour, we look at the data and find that the pigeon has pecked 24 times! It seems to be working. He seems to be *learning* that pressing the lever gets him something he wants.

We've proved our theory that if you follow a behavior with a reinforcer the behavior will occur more often.

Our little experiment has shown us something about the power of reinforcers. But what about that other kind of consequence, the punisher? What would happen if every time the pigeon pressed the lever, he got a shock of electricity through his feet (something we assume he doesn't like and would work to avoid)? The scientists ran the experiment. Sure enough; it worked. If the Behavior (pressing the lever) was followed by something the pigeon didn't like, the rate of lever pressing went down...until it went away all together. When a behavior stops occurring, that's called "extinction." The pigeon isn't extinct, but the behavior is.

Of course, this little story is a greatly simplified version of the kinds of experiments that took many years (and many graduate students) to perform. Gradually, our understanding of the role of reinforcers and punishers in shaping behavior became more sophisticated.

It wasn't long before the knowledge gathered in the animal labs was applied to people, particularly to people who have trouble learning new behavior. The technology of behaviorism arose just as the ICF-MR regulations began to require active treatment for all people with mental retardation. It seemed a perfect match. With the right rewards and punishers, it seemed we could teach anyone anything.

SOME ISSUES ABOUT REINFORCERS

In the next chapter, we'll get into how to use this research to teach people new skills. For now, let's spend a few minutes dealing with some of the trickier issues the researchers discovered when working with reinforcers.

IMMEDIACY

The first rule for reinforcers is that they work much more quickly if they immediately follow the behavior. If the pigeon pecked the lever and two minutes later a pellet dropped into the dish, it would be a long time before he connected the two events. His learning would be slower.

Of course, you and I don't seem to need to get our rewards immediately. You're probably used to working a week or a month before you get your paycheck. That's because you've already learned and understood the relationship between your work and the reinforcer. You can remind yourself that payday is the first and third Friday of each month and keep working. Someone who is learning a new skill for the first time, though, especially someone who doesn't have good language and understanding abilities, needs to have the reward right now. Not only does the reinforcer motivate the person to do the right behavior, it also serves as a signal that the job has been done. In most cases, the closer to the behavior the reward is given, the quicker the learning will occur.

You want to give the reinforcer immediately, but don't try giving the reinforcer first and expecting the behavior later. That's called "antecedent reinforcer" and if you've raised a child (or been one) you know that doesn't work.

You've seen this one in the grocery store. As Mom and little Joey enter the store, Joey starts screaming for some candy. Mom says, "OK, you can have some candy if you promise not to scream in the store." Of course, Joey agrees and he gets his candy. As soon as the candy is gone, what happens? Right—Joey starts screaming for more and he and Mom get into a shouting match about "listening." Doesn't Mom know that a three-year-old's contract is not legally binding? If Joey already has the reward, what motivates him to do the behavior? If Mom got some lessons in behaviorism, she would understand what the problem is. She would tell Joey that if he is quiet in the store, he will get a piece of candy *at the checkout*. First the behavior, *then* the reinforcer.

REINFORCER PREFERENCES

It's also important to remember that different people "like and will work for" different things. What motivates a person is called their "reinforcer preference." At Colin Anderson Center we had things we called "reinforcer aprons." These were cloth nail holders like you get at a building supply center. In each section of the reinforcer apron was a different edible reinforcer—cheese curls, raisins, peanuts, and the ever-present M&Ms. When we were going to do some training, we would tie on a reinforcer apron, load it with reinforcers from the locked reinforcer closet (staff were always lifting bags of cheese curls or corn chips for breaks), and away we'd go.

One day, Ruth, one of our better trainers, asked me for some assistance. She was training Patti to put on her shoes. When Patti finished the step she was working on, Ruth would attempt to put a "reinforcer" into Patti's mouth. No matter whether Ruth used peanuts, chips or the all-powerful M&M, Patti would spit them out, throw the shoe at Ruth and go on about her mysterious business. Ruth said to me, "I don't know how I can teach her anything if she won't take the reinforcer." A valid concern; but what was wrong with the statement? "She won't take the reinforcer" told me Ruth didn't truly understand what a reinforcer is. If something is going to function (operate) as a reinforcer (and make the behavior it follows more likely to occur again), it has to be "something the person likes and will work for." If Patti spit out the various items from Ruth's "reinforcer apron," it meant that these things didn't work as reinforcers for Patti. When you are trying to get someone to learn new skills and behaviors, be sure you have taken the time to find out what *she* likes and will work for. Otherwise, you're wasting both your time.

PRIMARY AND SECONDARY REINFORCERS

There's a trick to getting around having to know what each person's reinforcer preference is. See, most of the things we really like and will work for are what are called "primary" reinforcers. That is, they are things—like food and sleep and sex— that you don't have to learn to like. As a human being, you're hardwired to like those things. And most of us spend a good deal of energy working for them. Your employer, though, isn't going to come around on payday and give you the primary reinforcers of your choice. Instead, she's going to give a "secondary" reinforcer—something you had to learn the value of—money.

The nice thing about a secondary reinforcer is that when you receive it, you can decide what things you most want to trade it in for. You might spend yours on a new car payment, while I might use mine for books. Our employers can give us each the same reward, and we'll both keep working.

The drawback to secondary reinforcers is that you have to learn their value. I remember when Carl got his first paycheck from his first job. He'd never had money before, but he knew you needed it to buy things. He was very disappointed when he found out that his two five dollar bills didn't go very far at Circuit City. He had to learn how much of the secondary reinforcer he needed to trade for the primary reinforcers he really wanted.

Carl had mental retardation; it was hard for him to learn new things. So we didn't waste his time and ours teaching him to earn poker chips or points that he could trade for items at the "canteen." Those are institutional behaviors. Because we want Carl to have a life in the community, we teach him to use the secondary reinforcer we all use—money. Carl may never become the Chief Financial Officer at a Fortune 500 company, but he learned how much he needed for his weekly layaway payment on the stereo system he wanted. And that motivated him to keep working at his job.

SATIATION AND DEPRIVATION

One more thing about reinforcers. It involves a couple of words that are probably new to you, but don't let that throw you. You can amaze your family and friends by discussing them at the dinner table. What's important is that you understand the idea behind the words so you can avoid a common pitfall in using reinforcers.

The uncommon words are "satiation" (say-she-AY-shun) and "deprivation." Satiation looks a little like the word "satisfaction," and indeed it has a similar meaning. Satiation means to have enough, to be full, to be satisfied. Deprivation is just the opposite. It means to be deprived, hungry, not have enough.

These two are important to what we're talking about here because a person who has enough (satiation) of "something they like and will work for" is not going to be as motivated as someone who is hungry for that same thing (deprivation). If you need money to pay your bills and expenses (deprivation), your paycheck is important to you, and you're motivated to come to work and do a good job. But what would happen if you won $10 million in the lottery? You'd have "enough" (satiation), and you might think about going fishing instead of coming to work.

People who live in institutional environments often have all their basic needs met. It's hard to motivate them to work at a job if they've got "enough" for cigarettes, sodas and the occasional movie. You don't do a person any favor by rescuing him from his "deprivation." Being a little hungry for something never hurt anybody. It's what motivates most of us to get up off the couch.

I was excited when we were able to help Leslie move from the state hospital to a home with two other women. Leslie had mild mental retardation and bi-polar disorder. She wasn't very motivated. I said, "Leslie, one of the cool things we can do when you move to your new house is help you look for a job."

She replied firmly, "Oh, I don't want no job."

I said, "Yeah, but you know what happens if you don't have a job."

"Yeah; I won't have no money."

She was smarter than I thought. "But you know what happens if you don't have money," I said.

"Yeah," she responded quickly, "I'll have to go without."

I thought, "We're doomed. How are we ever going to motivate her to work if she feels like she already has enough?"

Fortunately, one of the staff people who worked with Leslie was a woman who had "water in her well." One afternoon, she took Leslie to the mall to look around. It was one of those off days at the mall, and a bored make-up artist offered to do a makeover for Leslie free. Leslie went for it. When she looked in the mirror, she really liked what she saw—especially the lipstick. When she found out how much that lipstick cost, she shook her head and pretended she didn't want it.

At another store, Leslie saw a purse she really liked. It cost $65. Leslie's coach told her if she was working she could save her money for a purse like that. Leslie shook her head and said, "I don't want no job."

Later that night, though, Leslie's hunger for those nice things must have grown. She was feeling deprived. She was ready to become a consumer (in the true sense of the word). She was also smart enough to know that if you want to be a consumer, you have to be a producer. The following morning, Leslie asked her coach if she could apply for a job. A little deprivation never hurt anyone.

THE ETHICS OF CONTROL

Leslie's reluctance to tell her coach how much she wanted the lipstick may have come from her institutional experience. She may have learned that whenever she told someone what she liked or wanted they would take it away from her and use it as a way to control her behavior. Be careful you don't do the same thing. Once we understand the power of reinforcers, it's tempting to use everything in a person's life as a way to make them behave the way we want them to. But people should be able to have some important things in their lives *regardless of their behavior.* Everyone has a right to positive attention, the opportunity to interact with others, a healthy diet, and time to be outside for exercise and fresh air. It is not right to withhold these things and make people earn them.

It is also considered unethical to use cigarettes as reinforcers. People become addicted to tobacco products (as you know if you smoke). An addict will do anything to get the fix he needs. Controlling someone's ability to get something he is addicted to gives you powerful control over the person. But it does not develop a relationship of equality that will help that person succeed in life.

THE PITFALLS OF PUNISHERS

I'll deal with the punishment issue more in Chapter 9, "Why Does She Act That Way?" For now, I just want you to think about the fact that human beings are not pigeons. Punishers often don't work on us the way they work on simpler creatures. We tend to rebel, to get mad, to try to get even. With people, punishers often make the situation worse rather than better.

Punishers don't motivate people or teach new ways of behaving. In short, though you need to know what a punisher is, I don't want you to put them in your bag of training tricks. We do better without them.

Let's go on to the next chapter now, and see how you can put your new learning to the test teaching people new skills.

Chapter 7

TEACHING REAL SKILLS FOR THE REAL WORLD

LEARNING TO GET ALONG IN THE WORLD

You need to know about how people learn and are motivated because you need to know how to teach people how to do new behaviors, behaviors that can be their ticket to a "Real Life in the Real World."

People who have mental retardation have trouble learning things. So it's important that the things we help them learn are skills that will help them get what they want out of life.

We all need skills in our daily lives. We need to know how to dress ourselves, keep ourselves clean, get the nourishment we need, find our way from place to place and get along with other people. We call these skills "adaptive behaviors." "Adaptive" means "helps you get along (adapt) in the world."

THE BEHAVIORIST APPROACH TO TRAINING

Most of the years I have been in this field, I have worked in programs that use the behaviorist approach to training. The behaviorist approach starts with "task analysis." Task analysis is taking a common adaptive task, say toothbrushing, and breaking it down into smaller steps. The smaller steps are supposed to make it easier for people who have trouble learning (people who have mental retardation).

Have you ever thought about the steps a simple task like brushing your teeth involves? Watch yourself some morning. It might seem to go something like this:

1. Put toothpaste on brush
2. Wet brush and paste
3. Brush teeth
4. Rinse mouth
5. Rinse brush
6. Put brush and paste away

But those are only the big steps. What does it mean to "put toothpaste on brush"? How do you do that if you have trouble learning new things? Well, you might break it down (analyze it) further. Step 1 might become:

1. Pick up toothpaste tube with left hand
2. Remove cap from tube with right hand
3. Place cap on sink
4. Pick up toothbrush with right hand
5. Place appropriate amount of paste on brush

You could do the same thing for each of the other five steps we started with. What you'd end up with is a 30-step task-analyzed toothbrushing program. Pretty intense.

How can someone who has trouble learning deal with such a complicated learning task? The technique the behaviorists came up with was called "backwards chaining." We would start with the last step in the program (Step 30, which might be "Put toothbrush away"). We would assist the person through the first 29 steps of the task then say, "Johnny, brush your teeth." Johnny would then put his toothbrush away, probably with assistance, and we would give him a reward—"Good job, Johnny." Notice that the reward comes at the end of the task (just where a reinforcer belongs).

Confused? So was everyone else—the trainers, the training program writers (like myself), and the people who were supposed to be learning new skills. Backwards chaining was an example of one of those things that works fine in the laboratory, but is just not the way people in the real world learn things. You probably didn't learn to brush your teeth through completing a 30-step task-analyzed toothbrushing program, did you? But during the behaviorist era, we thought people with disabilities needed special techniques to learn their way out of the institutions.

We were trapped in a cycle that didn't produce what we wanted (new skills in the people we were working with), but we were armed with research that "proved" these special techniques worked. So my colleagues and I spent endless hours writing programs, collecting and identifying data, revising programs, training and retraining staff, and changing reinforcers. Patti still didn't learn to put her shoes on.

The tragedy (I'm revealing one of my opinionated prejudices here—I told you I would) is that this kind of stuff continues today. The bureaucratic system of rules and regulations and procedures that has built up around funding is antiquated and teetering under its own weight. There are thousands of people working on endless training programs because people thought "the regulations require it." Actually, the regulations required that the training be "individualized" and relevant to the goals of the person being trained. But, as we have seen, the institutional mindset lends itself to everything being the same—and the individual gets lost in the shuffle.

The good news is that there are better ways to help people learn new tasks, and there are lots of people in the system who are advocating for those better ways. The regulations are changing; organizations are changing; the public attitude is changing. As a beginner, you have the opportunity to be part of a more successful future, one that really helps people with disabilities live real lives in the real world. You may work for an agency that still does things in the old way, and that will probably be frustrating for you if you see that it wastes everyone's time. But you can be part of the future if you can help bring about needed changes. Let's see what that future might look like.

INFORMAL TRAINING

Better than the formal training programs that are run in countless facilities around the world is an approach known as "incidental learning" or "informal learning." The idea of informal learning was developed by educators who observed how much children (and adults) learned from participating in activities that were not specifically "lessons." Maybe you or your kids have had an experience with this kind of learning in a classroom setting. The teacher sets up the task of building a replica of a colonial village. Everyone pitches in, has fun, and "incidentally" learns a lot about history, science, art and mathematics—not to mention how to cooperate with others in the completion of a task.

The word that is key to informal learning is *participation*. In informal learning, you learn by doing. You participate in an activity and learn by the fact of being involved.

Think about it. How did you learn how to clean your house? Did you take a class? Probably not. You probably helped a parent with the various chores and learned by observing, by trying things, by making mistakes. The behavioral principles still apply. Mom asked you to help (Prompt). You tried the task (Behavior). And you got praised for your successes (Reinforcer). It's just that you didn't learn the task through a formal program. You probably didn't even think of it as learning. It felt more like success, like doing a good job.

Some learning is "deliberate" (explicit). We are aware of it. "Oh, I just learned something." We tend to call it "knowledge." Another kind of learning is "accidental" (implicit). This is when we "get a feel for" something. We tend to call it "wisdom." I like to call the first "final exam" learning, and the second "riding a bicycle" learning. Interestingly enough, recent research has shown that "riding a bicycle" learning is done by a less developed part of the brain than the "final exam" kind. When people have developmental disabilities, the more complicated parts of their brains are usually the most affected. Thus, it makes sense that people who have developmental disabilities might learn things better through participation than by formal training.

We have seen, too, that people who live in segregated, "special" environments don't get to participate in a lot of the activities others in the community take for granted. They've been sitting in classrooms trying to learn the skills they need for being allowed to participate. You can see that this can become a trap—you learn skills by participating; but you're not allowed to participate until you've learned the skills.

APPLYING THE PRINCIPLES OF INCIDENTAL TEACHING

It's easy to say the best way to learn is by participating in the activity. But if you are a paid support professional, the powers that be are going to want to know what you are doing that is "training." You will need to be aware that there are some principles you should follow, rules of thumb that will make learning most effective.

People learn best when:
- they choose what activities they want to engage in
- the activities are from "real life"
- the skills are learned in the "real world"
- the task is participated in from beginning to end
- you "take what you can get closest to what you want"
- people are allowed to learn from mistakes
- you give only as much help as is needed
- you set up natural supports

Let's take a deeper look at these principles one at a time.

CHOSEN ACTIVITIES

It took me a long time to realize that shoe-tying was not something Patti was interested in learning. Though she used no words, she was constantly telling her trainers to leave her alone. She would hit a trainer over the head with the shoe, then run barefoot over to the window, pressing her face against the glass to see what was out there. What was Patti telling us? That she just wanted to go outside and get into whatever was out there. We said, in effect, "Patti, you can't go into the world unless you can tie your shoes." We weren't listening to her. We should have gotten her some loafers or some shoes with Velcro closures.

People (all people, including ourselves) learn best the things they really want to learn. The first principle of informal training is to pay attention to what the person wants to do. Even people who don't use words will communicate their desires to you if you pay attention. They will pull away from unwanted activities or just refuse to participate, but you'll have no trouble engaging their interest in a desired activity. When you know what the person wants to do, you then help her get involved in that activity. It seems like magic. All of a sudden she starts learning the things she needs to learn in order to do the thing she wants to do.

And using desired tasks for training gives the message that the person who is learning is the one who is in control. If you support people in choosing what kinds of activities they want to engage in, you will be sure that training is not an excuse for manipulative games, wasting both your time and theirs.

"REAL LIFE" ACTIVITIES

By "Real Life" I mean activities that are part of "Real Life in the Real World." When you're helping a person learn new skills through informal training, you should help her engage in activities that really need to be done, as opposed to tasks that are made up as training programs. A good question to ask is, "If Barbara (the person I'm supporting) wasn't doing this, would someone else have to?" That is, is it a necessary task or just a training game?

Old style special education is particularly guilty here. Classrooms, being removed from most of the stuff that goes on in the real world, don't have many real world tasks to get involved in. A typical example of the meaningless classroom task is "putting pegs in a pegboard." The student has to put colored pegs into rows of holes in a board. This is supposed to teach him such skills as color recognition, sequencing, attention to task, job stamina, following instructions, etc. The problem is that none of these things is something that really needs to be done. Putting pegs in a pegboard over and over, day after day, is boring, meaningless, and stupid.

Remember Our Standard— "Is this the kind of life I would like to live?" Would you like to spend a half hour putting pegs in holes, only to have the instructor come over to your table, say "Good job," then put the pegs back in the can and ask you to put them in the board again? Me neither. I might throw the pegs across the room and hit the teacher over the head with the pegboard. My actions would be saying, "I may be retarded, but I'm not stupid! Don't waste my time."

Is doing a pegboard a "Real World" activity? Just ask yourself whether the school would have to hire a Pegboard Technician II to make sure all the pegboards get done!

I was once asked to do my behaviorist thing in a "self-contained" (meaning "segregated") classroom for six children in the Severe and Profound range of mental retardation. They were kids who lived at one of the group homes I worked with. I had been asked to help with Chrissy, a 14-year-old girl who didn't speak and who had a reputation for very aggressive behavior when she didn't get her way. She was a lot like the Wild Boy of Aveyron you met in the history chapter.

When I got to the classroom and took my observation position in the back, the teacher was about to start the scheduled "music activity." This consisted of the teacher playing records, while the kids slept or rocked or wandered around the room. Chrissy did most of the wandering. I was counting how many times she was told to "Sit down and listen," when the phone rang in the teacher's office. The teacher went to answer it, telling Jerome, the Teacher's Assistant, to take over while she was gone.

Well, Jerome was as bored as the kids were, so he looked for something to do. He remembered that one of the chairs in the classroom had loose legs, so he decided to make the repair while the teacher was away. He went to the class toolbox, which was located on a high shelf, and got a screwdriver. As I realized what he was about to do, I said, "Jerome, I think Chrissy would like to learn how to fix a chair." Jerome looked at me like I had just spoken to him in Russian. "I'll help her," I said, and asked if I could borrow the screwdriver.

Chrissy had of course used the distraction as an opportunity to go see what was on the shelves. I called to her, "Chrissy, can you come over and help me with this chair?" She looked at me, wondering what I was up to (most of the attention she got was usually of the negative variety). As she approached, I said, "This is a Phillips screwdriver. See, we use it to tighten this screw." She watched me intently. "Do you want to try it?" I asked, and offered her the screwdriver. She took the screwdriver in hand and tried to match it up with the head of the screw. I gently guided her hands, and she let me help her turn the screw. When the chair leg was tight, I showed her that it was fixed and said, "Good job. Thanks for helping me fix this chair." Chrissy grinned, reached for the screwdriver, and indicated she wanted to tighten the other chairs. I could tell by the look on his face that Jerome understood what was going on. We had just engaged Chrissy in doing a "Real Life" task, and she learned it very quickly.

Unfortunately, the teacher didn't get it. After class, when I described what had happened while she was on the phone, her response was, "Jerome should have known better. Students are not allowed to use the tools." I bit my tongue.

LEARNED IN THE "REAL WORLD"

Similar to the rule about activities being "Real Life" is that they should be learned in the environment where they're going to be used—the "Real World." Because the special education teacher is usually stuck in the classroom, he has a hard time following this principle.

Do you have an ADL room in your home? Probably not. ADL stands for Activities of Daily Living, and the ADL room is a place in an institutional environment where there are fake kitchens and fake bedrooms where students can practice fake skills. Everyone then keeps their fingers crossed that the skills learned in the ADL room will be useful in the real world.

Applying a skill from one situation to another is called "generalization." The problem is that many people with mental retardation don't generalize very well. You teach Eric how to identify "community danger signs" as pictures on the table in the ADL classroom. Then you go out for a walk, and Eric wanders into the area behind the building that's clearly marked "Danger-High Voltage!" He hasn't generalized from the pictures on the table to the signs in the real world.

When you teach skills in a made-up "training" world, your students don't learn the real world skills they'll need for successful community living. There was a great example of this at one of the places I worked, a large state facility. The campus at this place was arranged with an access road that went all the way around the outside of the central cluster of buildings. In the back of the access road, there was a crosswalk painted on the road surface. At the edge of the crosswalk was a traffic light—red, yellow, and green. Do you think this traffic light and crosswalk were there because the traffic came whizzing by so fast that without it people would never get to the other side? Hardly. In fact, there wasn't even anything on the other side...just a field and some woods.

You've probably guessed its purpose by now. The crosswalk and traffic light were for teaching residents of the facility "pedestrian safety skills." A teacher would take a group of students out of the classroom (holding hands in a long chain—what I call "towing") and over to the crosswalk. She would then push the button to change the light colors, and say, "OK, it's safe to cross now." When they were finished with the lesson, the students would troop back to the classroom, having accomplished a little bit of "active treatment."

But did they learn anything they could use in the real world? If one of those students had the chance to walk around the middle of the little town that's a few miles from the facility, would he have understood the message of the stoplight and crosswalk at the town's main intersection? I think not. He wouldn't be able to generalize from one situation to the other. So what do we do?

I say we teach people community pedestrian skills in the community in which they'll be used. I'd like to see the teacher bring that class of adults from the state facility down to Main St. and learn right there. Not only would they not have to "generalize" their learning from one environment to another, but the real place also has many more cues you can learn from. The real intersection has, in addition to the stoplight and crosswalk, a flashing "Walk/Don't Walk" sign with a picture of a person walking or not walking. And it has other people walking or not walking. You could take your cue from them. And it has traffic either whizzing past or stopping while you cross. It may even have a helpful citizen who will sense your confusion and give you some assistance. But best of all, the real intersection has, down at the end of the cross street, a TCBY frozen yogurt store—a reason to cross the street! A built-in natural reinforcer!

Skills should be learned where they are going to be practiced. Learn job skills at the job site, not in "vocational training" classes. Learn social skills at a party or a dance. And learn dressing skills in the bedroom, while getting dressed to go out into the real world.

PARTICIPATE IN THE WHOLE TASK...
FROM BEGINNING TO END

In the section above, we looked at the task-analyzed, backward-chained way of teaching a new skill. One of the problems with that approach was that the person was only working on one "step" at a time. Sometimes she'd get stuck on a step, and we'd be pulling our hair out trying to figure out a way to get her to "pass" so she could get on with the task.

You can avoid this obstacle by always doing the entire task, from beginning to end. If you're helping a person learn to wash his clothes, the task starts with sorting the dirty clothes and ends with putting the clean clothes away. In between the beginning and the end, that particular person may quickly learn some of the steps of doing laundry (maybe measuring the soap) and have trouble with others (setting the dials on the machines). As you are helping him through the total task, he will be slowly learning all of the different sub-tasks at the same time. It's more fun. It's more meaningful (laundry does have to be done). And it's faster than the old tedious stepwise method.

Total task learning also has the effect of dealing with many "goals" at once. One day I was visiting one of the group homes I worked with, when Amy, a young woman with cerebral palsy who lived there, approached me in her wheelchair and said, "James, can I show you how good I'm doing on my dusting program?" I said, "Sure; I'd love to see how you're doing." Amy went to the staff person on duty and asked if she could do her dusting program for me. The staff person rolled her eyes (a capital offense in my rule book), looked at her watch (it was 4:00), and said, "Well, you're not supposed to do it until 4:30. But I guess we could." She (the staff person) then went to the utility cupboard, unlocked it, got out a can of dusting spray and a rag, brought the materials to an end table, wheeled Amy to the table, sprayed the table and handed Amy the rag. "OK, Amy," said the staff person, "Dust the table." Amy took the rag and made swirling motions with it on the surface of the table. "See how good I'm doing, James," she said with enthusiasm. I was not impressed.

The problem was that just two weeks earlier I had been at Amy's annual planning meeting. The physical therapist had said Amy's range of motion and upper body strength were worse than they had been the previous year. She said Amy needed to be encouraged to push herself anywhere she wanted to go in her wheelchair, and she prescribed stretching exercises Amy was supposed to do every day (at 4:45, when she finished her dusting program). The reason I was depressed was that I saw a lost opportunity. If Amy did the entire dusting by herself (or with only as much help as she needed), she would be working on her range of motion, her eye-hand coordination, and her physical stamina all at once. And she would be accomplishing this by doing something she obviously enjoyed doing (a chosen task) and that really had to be done (a "Real Life" task), in the place where it really occurs (her home). How much more mileage can you get out of one simple chore?

When I asked the staff person why Amy couldn't do the whole task, her first response was, "All the cleaning stuff is locked up. It's a rule." I suggested (as nicely as I could) that she could offer Amy the key to the cabinet. I know—it would be hard for Amy to hold the tiny key, fit it in the lock and get the door open. But it would help her develop her fine motor skill. And once she gets the cabinet open, where do you think I would like the dusting spray to be? That's right, just out of reach, so she has to stretch a little for it. And she should wheel herself to the table, take the cap off the spray, and push that little button. All of those tasks would be hard for Amy, but she's motivated. And if she doesn't use what skills she's got, she'll lose them. Let's give her the opportunity to develop everything she's got.

The second objection the staff person offered to Amy doing the entire task was, "It would take too long." See, the staff person, thinking of dusting as a "training program," was used to getting it "done" in 10 or 15 minutes. Then she would go on to another task, while Amy sat in her wheelchair in the living room and complained about what was on TV. Wouldn't it be better if Amy was busily engaged in trying to keep the house clean? So what if it took two hours? What else does Amy have to do?

Another Amy story: A few weeks after the episode with the dusting program, a different staff person at that home approached me and said, "I've found another way for Amy to work on her range of motion. She likes to load the dishwasher, and she has to lean across from her chair to reach the plates in the middle." That's the kind of creative approach I like. You go, girl!

TAKE WHAT YOU CAN GET CLOSEST TO WHAT YOU WANT

I said earlier that offering supports often requires patience. This is particularly true when you are teaching new skills. Sometimes a person's learning seems excruciatingly slow, but your job is to keep an enthusiastic attitude and motivate further achievement.

One way to build an attitude of patience into your professional repertoire is to learn the slogan "Take what you can get closest to what you want." It's a phrase that's been around for a number of years, and you'll be surprised at how often it is appropriate to your work.

"Take what you can get closest to what you want" is a layperson's expression of what behavioral psychologists call "shaping through successive approximation." I know, that's a mouthful, but when we break it down you'll see how useful an idea it is.

We've already used the word "shaping" with regard to teaching new behavior. It suggests that behavior is moldable and that it doesn't just leap from "now you don't know it" to "now you do." We shape behavior a little at a time by encouraging the person we're teaching to get a little closer to the ultimate goal with each attempt. That's what "successive approximation" means. "Successive" means one attempt after another. "Approximation" means not exactly what you want but something close. If each step is a little closer to the goal, you're making progress. And if you "take what you can get closest to what you want" you will be able to encourage the person you support to make progress in whatever size steps she is capable of making. You don't expect perfection every time. You just look for something that's a little closer than the last attempt.

Eddie was a young man who was prone to hit people when he was angry. I had been working with Eddie on what we called a "Safe Haven" program. When Eddie was upset, he was supposed to go to his Safe Haven (his bedroom) until he got himself together. One afternoon while I was in Eddie's home, he became very angry about something that was not going his way. He got up in my face and cocked his fist back as if he was about to punch me. I told him (verbal prompt) I thought he needed to use his Safe Haven to cool off a little. He hesitated, cursed me, stomped off to his bedroom and slammed the door. When he was calm, he came out and apologized. I told him I was very proud of what a great job he'd done using his Safe Haven. A staff person who was watching the interaction later told me she didn't agree with my response. "He cursed you and slammed the door," she said. "That's not good behavior, and you rewarded him for it."

I responded, "Cursing and slamming aren't perfect, but they're better than hitting me. His running off to his room was as close as he could get to what we ultimately want him to do. It was an improvement. So I took it."

If you will learn to reward people for their small steps in the right direction, their "successive approximations," you will find they are learning more than anyone ever thought possible. And you will be a great success.

LEARN FROM MISTAKES—THE OPPORTUNITY TO FAIL

A great part of growing into a life is learning which events, people, places, etc. are associated with good things happening and which with bad things. We then choose the good ones. Simple, right?

Well, maybe you're different from me, but I've certainly had times when it seemed terribly difficult to tell which decisions and actions were going to lead to good consequences (reinforcers) and which to bad (punishers). And I'm not talking about when I was a child. I'm talking about the way we live our lives as adults. We take risks. We make mistakes. Gradually, through sometimes painful trial and error, we learn. I've learned a lot more from my "failures" than I have from my "successes."

Why do we have the idea that people with disabilities don't also learn from their mistakes? There are a couple of reasons. One is that most people with disabilities have had lots of experience with failure. They've lived it; they understand it; they expect it. But they've had little experience with success. We want them to learn that they can be successful, so we try to minimize their failure.

Another reason is that service providers have taken responsibility for the lives of people with disabilities. Their failures become our failures. We don't want to fail, so we artificially protect them from the little failures we usually accept as lessons. And, more importantly, we take away their freedom to make choices in their lives. We can't allow them to choose something that will be a "wrong decision," because *we* are the ones who will suffer the consequences.

There is a problem with this approach. When we take the responsibility for people's lives we have to always be around, ready to cushion the fall. We know life is not like that. There are no cushion dispensers following us around. We have learned how to live by trial and error, with the loving support of family, friends, co-workers, neighbors. Sometimes it takes courage to make it on our own. It takes even more courage for people who have to overcome the obstacles of a disability. But courage is developed through engagement with life. We get out there and give it a try, and our parents and loved ones hope we don't fall too disgustingly on our faces. We learn by doing, by experimenting, and sometimes by asking others what their experience has been. We are rarely trained through a systematic application of rewards and punishments.

We need to turn people loose, give them the freedom to fail. We need to allow people with disabilities the opportunity to make the same kinds of non-fatal errors that have made us grow up and take responsibility for ourselves. I say "non-fatal" errors, because we certainly don't want someone to learn not to play in traffic by being hit by a truck. But, as the German philosopher Nietzche once wrote, "What does not kill me makes me stronger." If we help the people we support learn that they can take risks, make mistakes, and then pick themselves up and start over, we are helping them learn one of life's most valuable lessons.

GRADUATED GUIDANCE

The "take what you can get" philosophy uses reinforcers to shape new behaviors. It means you reward small successes that are closer to the ultimate goal. You can do the same kind of thing with Antecedents. You give only as much help as the person needs.

In the last chapter we talked about "prompts" as a form of Antecedent that causes a Behavior to happen. When training someone on a new skill, we want to use what is called a "prompting sequence." That means that when you want someone to do something you first Ask (verbal prompt), then Show (gestural prompt), then Assist (physical prompt).

You Ask Sally, "Sally, would you please put your glass on the counter?" Sally does not respond. She may be refusing to do what you asked, but she also might not understand the request. After giving her a chance to respond, you go to the next level of prompt. You Show (gestural prompt) Sally what you want her to do by acting out the behavior yourself. If Sally still does not respond, you have to decide whether she doesn't understand how to do the task or she is just refusing because she doesn't want to do it. If she doesn't understand how, you Assist her (physical prompt). You gently place your hand over hers and help her go through the motion of placing her glass on the counter. If she is refusing, you take a step back and try to understand what it is she wants to do.

The reason for using the different kinds of prompts in this order is that you want to encourage the person to do the task as independently as possible. Giving only as much help as the person needs or wants is sometimes called "graduated guidance." "Graduated" means adjusted to the situation. You have to become sensitive to the situation and to the person's ability and graduate your guidance so that your help is as light as it can be. This means giving a person time to respond to your request. It means using a light touch if you have to physically assist someone. It means staying behind the person, ready to offer help, but not leading the way.

Ultimately, we want to graduate our guidance right out of existence. This is sometimes called "fading." It means just what it says—our help fades away until it is no longer needed.

The goal of fading is to eventually become invisible as a support. Finally, we will see only the person, not the support or the support need— just as we want to make the wheel chair, or the hearing aid, or the white cane invisible. We all need supports for some things, but we don't want people calling attention to our need. The person who can't read may ask for help filling out an insurance form by saying, "I forgot to bring my glasses." The teenager who doesn't know how to deal with the lobster on her plate whispers under her breath, "How do you do this?" It is a sign of respect to offer assistance without making a big show of it. Paying attention to graduated guidance makes you sensitive to an important issue of providing support—give no less support than is needed and no more than is wanted.

SETTING UP NATURAL SUPPORTS

For years my work in the disabilities field centered on "Independence." It was even written like that, with a capital "I." When we wrote goals for training programs we used to write, "Terry will do such-and-such *independently*." Independently meant without help, without prompts, without support...completely on your own. People with disabilities were stuck in institutional environments until they could prove they could do everything Independently. Only then would they be let out to experience the world. It was sort of like the bank that won't lend you money unless you can prove you don't need it.

A few years ago, a new word started to arise—"Interdependence." Interdependence recognizes that none of us is Independent in the sense of needing no support or assistance from anyone. We all rely on a web of relationships with family, friends, co-workers, and neighbors to give us advice and help us in time of need.

The people in our personal life network are "natural" supports, in that they occur naturally in our lives, rather than being the result of a treatment plan or paid support program. "Real Life in the Real World" for people with disabilities expects them to have the same kind of network—and expects people to need support and assistance throughout their lives. Interdependence is universal; it applies to all.

It is important when you are teaching people new skills that you don't have the expectation that they will be able to do everything Independently. It is also important, however, that you help them set up the natural supports in their lives that will provide help with whatever things they aren't able to do by themselves.

Theresa had a job coach who helped her find a job that she liked and was successful at. The problem was the job was 20 miles away from Theresa's home. While the job coach, Debbie, was helping Theresa on the job, she also drove her to work every day. Debbie did a great job as a coach. She helped Theresa develop relationships with her co-workers. And she helped Theresa's co-workers learn how to offer Theresa the kinds of help on the job that Debbie had been providing. Finally, it came time for Debbie to "fade" as a job coach. Natural supports were in place at work, and Theresa no longer needed Debbie to be there.

But there was still the problem of transportation. Theresa was relying on Debbie for a ride to work. So Debbie started working on that part of the problem. She helped Theresa identify the bus route closest to her home where she could get a bus to work. She rode with Theresa for a couple of weeks, not only teaching Theresa which bus to take, how to buy her ticket, how to know when to get off, but also helping her get to know the bus drivers and other regular riders of that bus. With known people on the buses who she could turn to if she got confused or lost or scared, Theresa became confident enough to ride the bus without Debbie. She hadn't become Independent, but she had the natural supports in her life that allowed her to go beyond what paid supports can provide. Debbie had done a great job. She was able to turn her talents toward helping a different person with a disability learn as much as he could and rely on natural supports for the rest.

BE CAREFUL, TEACHER

Teaching people new skills that they have not had the opportunity to learn is a wonderful thing to do. It can open doors to new experiences and a sense of accomplishment for people who have had limited success in their lives. And while you teach you also learn. The teacher grows with her students.

But be careful you don't use your teacher role as an excuse to try to run someone's life for them.

Many people with disabilities have already spent many years being pushed around by The System. The old hospital/residential model, like Colin Anderson Center, encouraged a "do *for*" attitude. We took care of people, made their decisions for them, and kept them out of harm by segregating them from everyone else.

We made some progress when we moved to the training/habilitation model; but it quickly became a "do *to*" situation. We professionals felt entitled to train, program, assess, observe, and generally manipulate people with disabilities, because we thought they could *learn* their way into community inclusion. In our highly trained sophistication, we started to forget who should be the boss. Then we were surprised to find that a lot of people weren't appreciative of our efforts. They fought us for control, for the right not to learn, for the right to fail. Nobody wins that kind of struggle.

So, as you teach, use your best techniques, but remember to "do *with*." You are a partner with the person you support. You learn from the other person what his needs and desires and obstacles are, and he learns from you how to reach those goals and overcome those obstacles. "Doing with" is not only a more effective way for people to learn the skills they really need; it is also a much more satisfying way for you to work.

Chapter 8

MENTAL ILLNESS AND ITS TREATMENTS

Mental illness is different from mental retardation.

As we have seen in Chapter 5, mental retardation is a permanent characteristic of the way a person processes information about the world. It is not a disease that can be cured. For this reason, mental retardation is sometimes called a "trait" disorder. "Trait" means "a distinguishing quality or characteristic, especially of personality."

Mental *illness* is more like a disease that comes and goes. Sometimes the symptoms are better and sometimes they are worse. Mental illness is, therefore, called a "state" disorder. "State" means "a set of circumstances or attributes characterizing a person *at a given time*." We say, "Look at the state he's in."

Since they are different things, a person can have both mental retardation and mental illness at the same time. But our response to the two is often different. Mental retardation means the person will probably need some kind of lifelong *support* to be able to have a full and satisfying life. Mental illness, on the other hand, requires *treatment*, usually medication or therapy. With adequate treatment, the troubling symptoms of mental illness can often be reduced or eliminated. It is important for you to know about mental illness, as well as mental retardation, because some of the people you work with may have symptoms of both kinds of disorder.

MENTAL ILLNESS DEFINED

Just as we went to the panel of experts in AAMR for our definition of mental retardation, we will look to a group of expert psychiatrists to give us a definition of mental illness. This group, The American Psychiatric Association, publishes a book that is the chief reference text used by psychiatrists in the diagnosis of mental illness—*The Diagnostic and Statistical Manual of Mental Disorders-Version IV, 1994*—known more commonly as the "DSM-IV." The "IV" (four) is necessary, because this is the fourth manual of its type published since 1952. The reason for so many editions is that the experts' understanding of what mental illness is continues to change. Breakthroughs in knowledge about the brain and its chemistry and about the complex interaction of genetics, environment and experience are rapidly bringing progress to the understanding and treatment of the mental disorders that affect millions of people worldwide.

The definition of mental illness is not as clear and organized as the mental retardation definition was. The first part of the definition is that mental illness is "*a clinically significant behavioral or psychological syndrome.*" Let's take that one piece at a time.

"Syndrome" is a medical term that refers to a number of symptoms that occur together. A doctor needs to know all of the symptoms in order to come up with a diagnosis. One symptom, a headache for example, won't give enough information. But if your headache comes with itchy eyes and a runny nose, the doctor will probably diagnose your problem as allergies.

The "behavioral or psychological" part of the definition tells us that we are dealing with how the person acts (behavior) or how they think and feel (psychology).

"Clinical significance" means that the disorder being looked at causes "*significant distress or impairment in social, occupational, or other important areas of functioning.*" That is, the disorder is not merely an unusual personal style or a bit of strangeness. Rather, a "mental disorder" must be the cause of a level of distress and pain that becomes a major obstacle to the usual life tasks of the person.

This sounds a bit like the "difficulties in 2 or more life skills areas" phrase from the mental retardation definition, doesn't it? That's because the reason both mental retardation and mental illness are seen as problems is that they get in the way of a person experiencing a normally satisfactory life. Helping a person overcome these obstacles and get on with some kind of life is the main treatment goal, whether the person is dealing with mental retardation or mental illness or both.

Once it is established that the mental disorder is "clinically significant," it must then be determined that it is *not an expected response to an event*. For example, if a person's spouse of 40 years dies suddenly, we would not call her deep sadness and lack of appetite a "mental disorder"... unless it went on far past the time in which we would expect normal grief to occur. If a person were being mistreated and abused daily, we would not consider it mental illness that he was angry and defensive. Sometimes we respond to life events in ways that seem a bit "crazy" at the time; but if we then "get it together" and go on with our lives, no one is going to diagnose us as having a mental illness.

The final part of the definition gives you an idea of how large is the territory covered by "mental illness." Though the psychiatrists try to make a clear difference between "mental" and "physical" disorders, they admit that such a distinction is difficult. The mind and body are so intimately connected that many "mental" illnesses are found to have physical causes, and many "physical" illnesses have mental symptoms. Even so, we are talking about *illness* here, not just conflict or social deviance. A diagnosable mental disorder must be "*a manifestation of a behavioral, psychological, or biological dysfunction in the individual.*" "Dys-" means "something wrong" and "function" means "the normal or characteristic action of a thing." Something in the person is not working as it should and is causing strange behavior, strange thoughts, and difficulty functioning in the world.

Finding out whether that abnormal functioning is due to brain chemistry (the chemicals—neurotransmitters—that pass messages in the brain), brain physiology (how the brain is "wired"), or the fact that you had an overbearing mother is the hot research issue of the day. After all, the main purpose of diagnosis is the selection of the proper treatment. And we'll be able to select better treatments as we have better ideas about what causes the problems.

In review, then, mental illness is:
    1. a clinically significant behavioral or psychological syndrome,
    2. which causes distress, disability or an important loss of freedom,
    3. is not the expected response to an event
    4. and is the result of some sort of dysfunction.

Chapter 8 – Mental Illness and Its Treatments

MULTI-AXIAL DIAGNOSIS

Diagnosis is a difficult and challenging task. The word *diagnosis* comes from *dia*, meaning "between" and *gnosis* (NO-sis), which means "knowledge." Diagnosis is the process of deciding between two possibilities— *Is it This or is it That?*

An accurate diagnosis is crucial to deciding the correct treatment. If your doctor didn't notice the other allergy symptoms that went with your headache, she might send you for a CAT scan to see if you had a brain tumor—and you still wouldn't have medication to treat your allergies. Likewise with mental illness. Because of pharmaceutical breakthroughs in recent years, we have many effective treatments available to us. But you would be in a world of trouble if you had clinical depression and your doctor prescribed an anti-psychotic medication. Not only would you have to deal with the unwanted effects of the wrong medication, but your depression would go untreated.

Luckily, you don't need to make diagnoses. That's the physician's job. You will, though, be reading the medical records of the person you support, and you may be helping that person communicate with their doctor. It's important for you to know a little about psychiatric diagnoses.

The DSM-IV uses a "multi-axial" presentation of diagnoses. "Multi-axial" is a confusing term, but don't let it throw you. It just means that you will see several axis's, or "axes" (AX-eez), as they're more properly called. All you need to know is that when you look at a person's record, you will see something like this:

Axis I   295.90 Schizophrenia, undifferentiated type

        305.00 Alcohol abuse

Axis II 317 Mental Retardation, Mild

Axis III Hypertension

Each Axis addresses different kinds of disorders. Taken altogether, they make up the whole diagnostic picture:

- Axis I—Clinical Disorders (mental illness)
- Axis II—Personality Disorders and Mental Retardation

- Axis III—General Medical Conditions (like high blood pressure or diabetes)

- Axis IV—Psychosocial and Environmental Problems (e.g., living in a dangerous environment or with an abusive housemate; poverty; unemployment)

- Axis V—Global Assessment of Functioning (GAF) (this is a scale used to assess how serious the presenting problem is and then to track progress while in treatment)

The main difference between Axis I and Axis II is whether the problem is like an illness (Axis I) or like a personality characteristic (Axis II). It's what we talked about at the beginning of this chapter.

Axis I disorders are considered "state" conditions; that is, they are considered to occur from time to time (like an illness) and may be treated successfully for recovery or remission. Axis I conditions are most likely to be treated with medication, psychotherapy and/or hospitalization.

Axis II disorders, on the other hand, are "trait" conditions, expected to be lifelong, pervasive (affecting all areas of life), and chronic (being always present; not coming and going). Axis II conditions are more likely to be treated through long-term training and support programs. Some people believe the Axis II conditions are not really diseases and shouldn't be part of a diagnostic system.

The numbers in front of the diagnosis are a code used throughout the DSM-IV. You can look up 295.90 and get detailed information on what criteria are used to arrive at this particular diagnosis. And that's the best way to learn. Borrow someone's copy of DSM-IV (even in paperback, it costs $50) and look up the diagnoses you see on the record of the person you support. You may not understand all the terms and all the symptoms, but you'll at least become familiar with what the doctor is looking for.

PERSONALITY DISORDERS

In addition to mental retardation, Axis II is also the place for listing personality disorders. Personality disorders are strange critters, neither one thing nor the other. They don't seem to be due to a dysfunction in the brain or nervous system, like mental retardation and mental illness are, but they sure cause a lot of difficulty having a successful life.

All of us have personalities, preferred ways of dealing with life. A personality becomes a "disorder" when it:
- "deviates markedly from the expectations of the individual's culture" (DSM-IV)
- is "pervasive," meaning it affects all areas of the person's life
- is "inflexible," meaning the person's style of relating doesn't adapt to different circumstances
- and "leads to distress or impairment." It's not just eccentric; it causes the person and those around him pain and grief.

The DSM-IV lists ten types of personality disorder:
- Paranoid—distrustful and suspicious
- Schizoid—detachment from relationships and restricted range of emotional expression
- Schizotypal—acute discomfort in close relationships, cognitive or perceptual distortions, and eccentric behavior
- Antisocial—disregard for and violation of the rights of others
- Borderline—instability in relationships, self-image, and mood; impulsive
- Histrionic—excessive emotionality and attention seeking
- Narcissistic—self-centered, lacks empathy for others
- Avoidant—hypersensitive to criticism, feelings of inadequacy
- Dependent—submissive, clinging, excessive need to be taken care of
- Obsessive-Compulsive—preoccupied with orderliness, perfection, and control

BASIC CLASSES OF MENTAL ILLNESS

There are many types of mental illness. The DSM-IV lists 16 major "classes" or types of disorder, with over a hundred actual diagnostic categories. You would need a lot of clinical training to fully understand all of them. All I'll do here is give you an overview of the kinds of things you will find in the records of the people you support. It will be up to you, then, to learn more about a specific condition or illness.

The chart below shows you some of the classes, or types, of mental illness you will run into, along with the names of a few of the specific disorders that fall within each class, and some of the symptoms you would be expected to see. It's only a very brief summary, but it should give you the lay of the land. If you have trouble with any of the terms, you can look them up in the Glossary in the back of the book. If the person you are supporting has a particular diagnosis, you can get more information about it from the sources listed in the Resources section. There are lots of information sources designed for family, friends and supporters of people who have mental illness. You don't need any formal training to understand them. Be your own teacher.

SOME TYPES OF MENTAL DISORDERS—AXIS I

Class	Specific Disorders	Symptoms
Delirium, Dementia, Amnesia	Alzheimer's Vascular Substance-induced HIV	Disturbances of thinking and memory, short or long duration
Substance Related Disorders	Various substances	Depends on the substance and stage of addiction/use
Psychotic Disorders	Schizophrenia Schizoaffective disorder Atypical psychosis	Delusions Hallucinations Disorganized speech or behavior
Mood Disorders	Depression Bi-polar disorders	Disturbance in mood, attitude, behavior
Anxiety Disorders	Panic attacks Phobias Obsessive-compulsive disorder (OCD) Post-traumatic stress disorder (PTSD)	Apprehension, fearfulness, worry, compulsive behavior, flashbacks of stressful events

SOME TYPES OF MENTAL DISORDERS—AXIS II

Class	Specific Disorders	Symptoms
Mental Retardation	Mild Moderate Severe Profound	Sub-average IQ Occurs before age 18 Related difficulties in life skills areas
Personality Disorders	Borderline Paranoid Anti-social Narcissistic Dependent	Stressful, enduring pattern of behavior which deviates from cultural expectations, is inflexible and pervasive

DUAL-DIAGNOSIS

If you review the definitions you've just learned, you will see that mental retardation and mental illness are two very different types of condition. Mental retardation is a developmental disability that slows a person's ability to understand and use information. Mental illness, on the other hand, takes various forms, can occur at any time during life, and affects perception (what the world looks like) and emotion (how a person feels about what happens). Does it make sense that a person could have both mental retardation and mental illness? Yes, of course it does. We call this combination "dual-diagnosis."

Some clinicians are uncomfortable with this term because it means different things to different people (therefore, possibly not meaning anything at all). For instance, many psychiatric clinicians use "dual-diagnosis" to refer to someone who has both mental illness and substance abuse issues.

The recognition of "dual-diagnosis," that people with mental retardation can also have mental health needs that can be treated, is one of the most important realizations of the last half of the 20th century.

It used to be thought that people with mental retardation were not "smart enough" to have depression, but studies done in the 1980's showed that people who have lived in institutional environments may in fact have depression at many times the rate of the general population. The depression was not diagnosed because all people saw was the mental retardation. With our understanding that people with mental retardation are fully human, we have come to appreciate that they are subject to all of the problems we humans can have, including mental illness.

The publisher of this book is an organization that specializes in addressing the issues of dual-diagnosis: *NADD—An association for persons with developmental disabilities and mental health needs* (formerly National Association for the Dually-Diagnosed). Some of the issues brought to the fore by the pioneering clinicians associated with NADD are:

1. How do you get an accurate diagnosis for someone whose communication skills are limited?

2. Given that "disorganized thinking" is a symptom of both mental retardation and psychotic illness, how do you tell which is which?

3. How do you monitor the effects of treatment in a person who has little self-awareness and can't report on the progress of symptoms?

4. What are the interactions of various mental illnesses and developmental disabilities, interactions that can cause "atypical" (not what's usually expected) presentations?

5. How do psychotropic medications work differently in people whose central nervous systems are functioning differently from normal?

It is important to make the distinction between mental retardation and mental illness, because there is no truly *medical* treatment for mental retardation. And from this realization that mental retardation is not the same thing as mental illness, we get the second most important notion for our field—that people who have mental retardation are not sick...unless they are. There is no drug that can treat "significantly sub-average intellectual functioning." There are, however, good medications and therapies to treat a number of mental illnesses.

Mental illnesses require "treatment," whereas developmental disabilities require "habilitation," which consists of education, training and support. We'll look more at the issues involved in habilitation in later chapters.

Knowing what conditions are present and what treatments are appropriate is the job of a well-trained and sensitive medical practitioner (doctor, nurse, therapist). But you need to know about these differences, so you can be a better advocate for the people you support.

Remember the old "medical model?" It still tries to put doctors and nurses in charge of the lives of people who need support and training rather than medical treatment. I strongly advocate that medical clinicians be involved only in the treatment of diseases (Axis I and Axis III) and leave the task of helping someone overcome handicaps to social support people like you and me.

MIS-DIAGNOSIS = MIS-TREATMENT

One interesting research finding regarding dual-diagnosis is that people who have mental retardation are more likely to be diagnosed by psychiatrists as having a psychotic illness (schizophrenia, schizoaffective disorder) than as having an affective (mood) illness, like depression or bi-polar disorders. People who have mental retardation who live in institutional environments often act in strange ways that look like the bizarre behavior seen in people who have mental illness. When you're a psychiatrist with limited knowledge of the patient, it's easy to misinterpret what you see.

It often works something like this. Tony comes into the psychiatrist's office accompanied by Jeff, a staff person at the group home where Tony lives. The doctor asks Tony how he is feeling. Tony starts into a rambling report about something the doctor doesn't understand. The doctor asks Jeff what's going on with Tony. Jeff says sometimes Tony doesn't want to do anything. He just sits around and mumbles repeatedly about stuff the staff can't understand. And last Wednesday, the night everyone in the group home goes to the mall, Tony refused to go, then broke one of his windows and threatened to kill someone with the broken glass. Jeff says Tony keeps talking about "crazy stuff" that doesn't have anything to do with the activity at hand. He adds that two staff have already quit because of Tony's violent threats and they desperately need the doctor to do something.

The doctor concludes that Tony's incomprehensible mutterings may stem from hallucinations or delusions and that his unwillingness to participate in enjoyable activities may be due to an underlying depression. He makes a "Provisional" (tentative) diagnosis of "Schizoaffective disorder" and prescribes a medication for that condition. He tells Jeff to watch Tony and come back in a month. Jeff is satisfied, because he believes the "meds" will make Tony better behaved at the group home. The problem is that the diagnosis was made on very little information. If it's wrong, Tony won't get any better and could actually get worse.

Now, that scene is not how it always goes. Many courageous and caring psychiatrists work very carefully to try to understand the often strange world of a person with mental retardation and mental health needs. But they work under constraints of time set by Medicaid, HMO's and overbooked schedules. And some of them just don't have much training in dealing with developmental disabilities. That's why it's important for you to know about the diagnoses and medications that are being applied to the person you support. You can advocate for her, interpret for her, help her understand and recognize any side effects that come from the medication. And you can help the doctor by bringing clear reports of what's going on with her, and keeping records of any change in symptoms. When social support people and medical people work together in a creative partnership that has the patient at the center, miracles are worked.

Take the case of a woman I'll call Esther. When I first met Esther, she was living in a locked ward at a state-operated psychiatric facility. She spent most of every day lying in her bed in a fetal position, wouldn't talk to anyone, and wouldn't eat. She had daily tantrums. She wouldn't wear clothes, though staff could sometimes get her to wear a housecoat. When she "got mad," she would masturbate frantically, while screaming and crying. When these episodes occurred, Esther was put into four-point restraints, her wrists and ankles tied to the corners of the bed. When she wouldn't eat, she was fed with a tube through her nose into her stomach. She had been given a laundry list of medications, sometimes 3 or 4 at a time. It was my job to help her move into a home in the community.

I had been working with a private practice psychiatrist I'll call Dr. Smith, who had been seeing several of the people who lived in the other group homes I worked with. He was very attentive to our people and was willing to work collaboratively with me to find the best treatment in these often puzzling cases.

I wanted Dr. Smith to see Esther as soon as she moved into her new home. I had seen great results from a new medication, risperidone (Risperdal), and I wanted to see if Dr. Smith thought we should try it with Esther. Esther, however, would not get dressed to leave the house and made it known plainly that she was not interested in seeing "no GD doctor."

After a couple of weeks, one of the women who worked at Esther's home was able to get Esther to ride in the van. So we made an appointment for her to see Dr. Smith. I was at Dr. Smith's office the night of Esther's appointment, assisting several of the people who lived in our other homes. The staff person from Esther's home came into the waiting room and told me Esther was in the van in the parking lot but was loudly refusing to come into the doctor's office. I knew Dr. Smith would not prescribe anything without seeing Esther, but Esther was not willing to see Dr. Smith. So I went back inside the office and asked Dr. Smith if he would come out to the parking lot and see Esther there. He said he would (it pays to a have a good relationship with the psychiatrist).

After seeing how agitated Esther was and hearing about how she acted at the group home, Dr. Smith made a tentative diagnosis of Schizoaffective disorder and agreed to a trial of Risperdal. The medication would be started the next day, and Dr. Smith wanted to see Esther again in two weeks.

As the two weeks passed, there were reports from Esther's staff that she was settling down some, was more willing to engage in activities and was having fewer tantrums. When the appointment with Dr. Smith came, I was looking forward to seeing any signs of improvement. What happened exceeded my wildest dreams. I walked into the waiting room of Dr. Smith's office and there sat Esther. She was dressed nicely in a new skirt and blouse, sitting calmly, holding a new pocketbook in her lap. When I entered the room she looked up and said, "Hello, James"— the first time she had ever greeted me by name. The staff person said, "Esther, tell James what you're doing tomorrow." She replied, "Start my new job." You could have knocked me down with a feather.

Some of the people we support, people like Esther, face the dual challenges of mental retardation and mental illness. It has been very difficult for them to be successful in life. But with the right combination of accurate diagnosis, good psychiatric treatment, and adequate support, training, and opportunity, many of these people can lead productive, interesting lives.

PSYCHOTROPIC MEDICATION

In recent years, the treatment of mental illness has come more and more to rely on the use of psychotropic medication. The word "psychotropic" comes from the root *psycho*, which refers to the mind, and *tropic*, which means "alteration or change." A psychotropic substance, therefore, is anything which alters (changes) thinking, feeling, or behavior.

Can you think of a substance that meets this definition but is illegal? Certainly—cocaine, marijuana, LSD—most of the various illicit drugs are psychotropic. How about substances that are legal and require no prescription? You may be a user of some of these. Caffeine is my favorite, but you may prefer nicotine or alcohol. All of these substances alter thinking, feeling, and behavior. They are all psychotropic.

When we talk about psychotropic *medication*, we are limiting ourselves to those substances which are prescribed by a physician for the treatment of some disease or disorder.

We are treading on dangerous ground here. For many years, in institutional placements for people with mental retardation, powerful psychotropic medications were used to control people's behavior. It was called "chemical restraint." People who had "behavior problems" were given daily doses of Thorazine or Mellaril or Haldol (antipsychotic medications). These drugs are appropriately used to limit hallucinations and delusions in people who have psychotic disorders, but they are also powerful tranquilizers. They turned people into walking zombies, easier to manage, but no longer themselves. Give an agitated person a shot in the butt of 5 mg. of Haldol (what emergency room staff sometimes refer to as "Vitamin H"), and they will usually settle down and stop being a danger to themselves or others. But long term use of these medications as a restraint is an inappropriate intervention. Not only do these medications have long-term damaging side effects, but the agitation may not be caused by mental illness at all. As you will see in chapter 9, people in institutional settings often act badly because they are treated badly. Medicating them to settle them down does not address the real issue.

It is now considered bad practice, if not abuse, to use medication *in place of* appropriate treatment and support. But it was once done so commonly that a backlash reaction set in. Human rights committees and governing boards started *prohibiting* the use of psychotropic medications in people with mental retardation. People who had been on powerful drugs for years were suddenly taken off of them in support of their "rights." And people who needed the medication for the treatment of a properly diagnosed mental illness were not allowed to get it. Sometimes these ill-considered acts had devastating consequences (see Tommy's story below).

What is needed is a balanced, systematic approach to the use of medication. This approach must be:

- responsive to the needs of each individual patient
- based on observation
- supported by a caring team of professionals, family and friends

THE MEDICATION PROCESS

As a member of the support team of the person you are working with, you can help him through the process of making sure he is taking:

- the right drugs (for a correctly diagnosed condition)
- in the right amounts

The first step in this process has been discussed above—diagnosis. By helping assure that the physician gets good information about symptoms, behavioral changes, and any other aspect of the person's life the doctor feels is relevant, you can help the diagnostic process.

Once a good diagnosis is made, the doctor will prescribe a plan of treatment. This plan should always be empirical (em-PEER-i-cull), which is to say, based on observation of the patient's response. Medications should be changed or added one at a time, and enough time should be allowed for the patient to adjust to the change.

Your observation of the person taking the medication is important because the doctor may be working on a diagnostic hypothesis (high-PAW-thuh-sis). That's an educated guess that needs to be tested. Let's say the doctor's diagnostic hypothesis, based on the symptoms she sees, is that the person has depression. She prescribes an anti-depressant medication on a trial basis. You will be helping in the process of observing:

1) Is the medicine having the desired effect? Is it reducing the symptoms that are being addressed?

2) Is the medicine having any undesired effects? (See "An Aside on Side-effects," below)

If the person you are supporting has difficulty giving the doctor information about what's bothering him, the doctor will rely on you for this information. Make sure you are as accurate as possible. Don't exaggerate troublesome behavior because you believe it will make the doctor give the person medications. Let the doctor evaluate the information, make the diagnosis, and suggest the treatment. Your job is to supply information that is accurate, complete and respectful of the person you are supporting.

You may be asked to collect data (information) about behavioral outbursts, evidence of hallucinations or delusions, appetite, sleep patterns, strange movements, or anything else the physician thinks is relevant. You should be sure to ask the doctor what kinds of side effects the medication might have. Make sure what you are supposed to observe is accurately described in a way that everyone can agree on what is seen. You will need to describe these things to your co-workers in a way that everyone works together. *Collecting accurate data and reporting it clearly is an important part of the medication process.* Together with the physician, the rest of the team, and the patient, you can help a person overcome a sometimes-longstanding obstacle of mental illness.

HUNDREDS OF NAMES; THOUSANDS OF PILLS

The world of psychotropic medication is a bewildering maze, even for the clinical professionals who deal with these drugs every day. These medications usually have both a generic name (e.g., thioridazine) and a brand name (e.g., Mellaril). Each pharmaceutical company comes out with its own, slightly different, version of something proven effective. And there are new medications in clinical trials and coming onto the market almost every day. It would be impossible for me to teach you all of this or for you to keep up with the changes. So I'll again just give you a feel for the territory and point you in the direction of finding more information for yourself.

Medications are usually separated into classes, according to the type of disorder they treat; though new research is showing that drugs developed for one kind of illness are now proving to be effective with something else. So take the chart at the end of this chapter as a very oversimplified map of the territory.

SOME CLASSES OF DRUGS AND THEIR USES

ANTIPSYCHOTICS

We'll start with antipsychotic medications, since they have the longest history and will be seen very often in your work. Antipsychotic medications reduce the symptoms of psychotic illnesses like schizophrenia. This is a tough job, because there is no clear agreement on what causes these symptoms. What is agreed is that people with psychotic illnesses are often tortured by visions of reality that don't correspond with what you and I usually see (hallucinations). They hear voices or sounds inside their heads; they smell strange odors; they interpret events as being directed toward them in frightening ways (delusions, paranoia); or they have bouts of withdrawal or rage or inappropriate laughter. Antipsychotic medications can reduce these symptoms enough that the person can start getting their life back together.

Chlorpromazine (Thorazine) was one of the earliest antipsychotic medications. Developed in the 1950's, it seemed like a miracle at the time. Patients who had spent much of their time screaming, restrained by leather straps, became calm and quiet. This was the first of a group of drugs that work on the neurotransmitter Dopamine. Later developments in this group were thioridazine (Mellaril), haloperidol (Haldol) and fluphenazine (Prolixin). All of these medications give some relief from the hallucinations and delusions that plague someone who has a psychotic disorder. But they also share some serious side effects.

A number of new antipsychotic drugs (the so-called "atypical antipsychotics") have been introduced since 1990. The first of these, clozapine (Clozaril), has been shown to be more effective than other antipsychotics, although the possibility of severe side effects — in particular, a condition called agranulocytosis (loss of the white blood cells that fight infection) — requires that patients be monitored with blood tests every one or two weeks. Even newer antipsychotic drugs, such as risperidone (Risperdal) and olanzapine (Zyprexa), seem to be safer than the older drugs or clozapine, and they also may be better tolerated.

New antipsychotics are coming onto the market all the time. You may have to check into one of the websites listed in the Resources section at the end of this book for the latest information.

AN ASIDE ABOUT SIDE EFFECTS

Side effects are enough of an issue with psychotropic medication to warrant a little aside about them. Bear with me a few minutes, and we'll get back to the classes of medications.

Medications often do things that, just because they're not the *desired* effects, are written off almost casually as "side effects." Don't you find it amazing, now that the pharmaceutical companies are allowed to advertise on TV, that the "side effects" of a drug are often just like the disease that's supposed to be treated? For instance, a remedy for chronic heartburn "may cause upset stomach, nausea or diarrhea." Oh, well; I won't worry about those. They're only "side effects."

The side effects issue becomes even more critical when you're dealing with psychotropic medications. Psychotropic medications are powerful stuff. They work on critical parts of the nervous system, sometimes in ways that are not completely understood. Some of the "side effects" of commonly prescribed psychotropic medications include confusion, agitation, insomnia, dizziness, and fatigue. These are bad enough if you understand what's going on. But suppose you have mental retardation and you don't really know why you're feeling so bad? Might you not "act out" in inappropriate ways?

It is part of your job to know all of the effects of the medications the person you are supporting is taking. Do your homework. You may be able to help the person you support talk to their doctor about the possibility that the bad feeling they are having is from the medication. Or the physician may not realize the severity of these effects, because he doesn't know the patient as well as you do. Or the person may be refusing to take the medication, unable to explain why, when the real reason is that it just makes him feel bad.

One common group of side effects is caused by the anticholinergic (*ant-ee-cole-in-urge-ic*) action of many medications. Among these anticholinergic effects are:
- dizziness

- dry mouth
- constipation

Sometimes these are tolerable, given the beneficial effect of the medication; and a person's doctor can help him learn how to deal with them. At other times, the patient ends up getting more medication to deal with the side effects, and the effects keep mounting on top of each other. Anticholinergic effects also make it very difficult to stop taking some medications. *Never advocate for a person to stop their medication or change their dose without an order from their physician.*

More serious is a long-term effect of some anti-psychotic drugs (the ones we were looking at when I started this aside). Called tardive dyskinesia, the name comes from *tardive* (TAR-div), meaning "late onset" and *dys (dis)*=bad and *kinesia* (kin-EE-zsuh)=movement. It is, therefore, *a late onset movement disorder*, presenting symptoms of facial grimacing, random chewing movement, and uncontrolled movement in head, arms and legs. It is neither curable nor reversible. Once it shows up, the damage has been done. It is caused by long-term use of some antipsychotic drugs. You will probably learn more about how to watch for its symptoms (usually through the use of the AIMS—Abnormal Involuntary Movements Scales) in your medication training class.

EPS or extrapyramidal (ek-stra-pi-RAM-i-dul) symptoms can look similar to those of tardive dyskinesia, but they may occur even after a few doses of a medication. These include acute dystonia (spasms, drooling, difficulty breathing), pseudoparkinsonism (tremor, rigidity, drooling, shuffling gait), and akathisia (restlessness, agitation).

Once again, it is critical that you know the side effects of any medications taken by the person you are supporting. Help him/her learn what they are, too. Together, you can keep the person's physician informed, to make sure the person is taking the right dosage of the right medication for them.

BACK TO THE CLASSES OF DRUGS

ANTIDEPRESSANTS

The next class of psychotropic medications to be considered is the antidepressants. These are used to treat depression (and sometimes other conditions, such as Obsessive-Compulsive Disorder). Someone who is treated appropriately with antidepressant medication should expect to have more energy, a more positive attitude, and better eating and sleeping patterns. An older generation of antidepressants (known as "cyclic" drugs) have good positive effect on depression but commonly produce anticholinergic side effects and weight gain. Recently, a new class of medication, the SSRI's (Selective Serotonin Reuptake Inhibitors) has revolutionized the treatment of depression and other emotional disturbances. The most commonly known SSRI, Prozac (fluoxetine), has become one of the most widely prescribed drugs in America. Others include Zoloft and Paxil. The SSRI's can take several weeks to take effect, so it is important to help the person taking them to stick with them long enough to give the medication a fair trial. They are also much more expensive than the older anti-depressants, which recent research has shown work just as well.

ANTIANXIETY AGENTS

The Antianxiety Agents are used in the treatment of panic attacks, phobias and Obsessive-Compulsive Disorder. These make a person feel calmer and less fearful. Many of these medications are in a chemical class known as benzodiazepines. Though they are very effective for short-term treatment, they are highly addictive. They may also cause falls and confusion in elderly patients.

Many antianxiety drugs make people feel so good that they are commonly self-administered by people who do not have prescriptions for them. For this reason, most of these medications are Federally Controlled Substances and have to be administered under strict guidelines to prevent abuse.

ANTI-CONVULSANTS

Some medications that were originally prescribed for the control of seizure disorders were found to have mood-stabilizing effects. They are often used for people who have the mood swings that are characteristic of Bi-polar disorders.

OTHER MEDICATIONS

Finally, some medications that were originally intended for control of blood pressure and heart rate (Beta blockers) were found to have a calming effect on people who had panic attacks, explosive disorders and mood swings.

As I said above, this is a very simple introduction to psychotropic medication. You will have to study on your own to learn more about the medications the person you are supporting is taking. You can refer to patient information sheets that come from the physician or pharmacy, layman's manuals like those listed in the Resources section of this book, or pharmaceutical and patient advocacy sites on the Internet.

A CAUTIONARY TALE

Let me close this chapter with a story that illustrates the need for knowledge about mental illness, medications, and proper medication process.

Tommy was a 27-year-old man who lived in a group home with five other people. He had lived many years in a state psychiatric facility and had the reputation of being very aggressive and disruptive. His first few months in a community-based group residence with 5 other people were largely uneventful. Tommy liked the additional social contact the new home provided, and he was often helpful with the less capable residents. During the course of his treatment planning, I expressed some concern that he was taking Phenobarbital, a powerfully addictive barbiturate. His medical record (which is generally incomplete in cases of long-term institutionalization) mentioned "a history of seizures" going back many years. Since Phenobarbital used to be used as an anticonvulsant (seizure control) medication, it seemed reasonable that that's why he was taking it. But in talking with his mother one day, she said he had only had one seizure "when he was a little boy," and that the Phenobarbital had been prescribed in the hospital because of Tommy's aggressive outbursts, an inappropriate chemical restraint.

We set up an appointment for Tommy to see the neurologist to evaluate whether he needed to take the Phenobarbital to control seizures. Two days after the neurology appointment (which I couldn't attend because of a schedule conflict), I received a frantic phone call from one of the group home staff. She said Tommy had "gone crazy" and was running around the home yelling at people for no apparent reason. He had already bitten two of his housemates, one of them rather badly. I went to Tommy's home right away, and, sure enough, he wasn't himself. He looked at me slyly and wouldn't make eye contact. His breathing was irregular, and his face looked flushed. I asked the staff what they thought had caused this sudden change. They all said it happened "right after we stopped the Phenobarbital." Alarm bells went off in my head. I had not been told the results of the neurologist appointment. Now I found out that the doctor said Tommy did not have seizures, and his Phenobarbital should be discontinued immediately. The nurse had made the change in the medication record without consulting the other members of Tommy's team. As a result, Tommy was in full-blown withdrawal from a powerfully addictive drug he had been taking for many years.

I called the nurse on call, and she reached the doctor, who ordered reestablishment of the Phenobarbital at half the original dose (he said no one had told him how long Tommy had been on the Phenobarbital). This should have helped Tommy withdraw more slowly. It didn't. He continued to bite people and agitate everyone in the house. It took another six months for Tommy to get back to his old self.

This was a powerful lesson in why these kinds of decisions must be made by a group of people. Doctors who don't know their patients very well can make mistakes. They are relying on us for good information and as a questioning safeguard. So it is important that you learn all you can about the medication a person you are working with is taking. Learn what it is usually prescribed for and what the usual dose is. Learn its side-effects, both long-term and short-term. And help the person you support talk with the doctor so that medical decisions are made in a collaborative way, the same way you'd like your doctor to work with you.

SOME CLASSES AND EXAMPLES OF PSYCHOTROPIC MEDICATION[1]

Class		Generic	Brand name
Antipsychotics	Older Generation	fluphenazine	Prolixin
		haloperodol	Haldol
		chlorpromazine	Thorazine
		thioridazine	Mellaril
		molindone	Moban
		thiothixene	Navane
	Newer Generation	risperidone	Risperdal
		clozapine	Clozaril
		olanzipine	Zyprexa
		quetiapine	Seroquel
Antidepressants	Older Generation	desipramine	Norpramin
		imipramine	Tofranil
		amitryptiline	Elavil
		trazodone	Desyrel
	Newer Generation	paroxetine	Paxil
		sertraline	Zoloft
		fluoxetine	Prozac
		clomipramine	Anafranil
		mirtazapine	Remeron
Antianxiety agents		diazepam	Valium
		lorazepam	Ativan
		alprazolam	Xanax
		hydroxyzine	Vistaril
Seizure drugs[2] (anti-convulsants)		carbamazepine	Tegretol
		divalproex sodium	Depakote
		clonazepam	Klonopin
Other		lithium[3]	Eskalith, Lithonate
		buspirone	Buspar[4]
		propranolol	Inderal

[1] Regarding pronunciation: You will hear lots of different pronunciations, even from the clinical professionals who work regularly with these medications. Listen to them, and use the pronunciation that seems to be most common where you work.

[2] Sometimes used for mood stabilization.

[3] Lithium is not technically a drug, but a naturally occurring mineral salt. It is used for treatment of bi-polar disorder.

[4] Buspar and Inderal are commonly used to treat blood pressure and heart rhythm problems but have also been found to have some positive effect in certain anxiety conditions.

Chapter 9

"WHY DOES SHE ACT THAT WAY?" —UNDERSTANDING CHALLENGING BEHAVIOR

"BE GOOD, BE GOOD, BE GOOD."

Though I met Walter when he was an adult, I learned from his mother that he had been a handful his whole life. She told me about the time she came in from picking beans in the garden and six-year-old Walter had pooped in his pants, then painted the dining room walls with it. Even at age six, Walter was not toilet trained and could not speak more than a few barely understandable words.

Walter's mother told me about the episode that led to Walter being "sent away" when he was nine years old. He got mad about something and cleared the pantry shelves of canned goods, throwing the cans through the windows of the house. Mom left the house, afraid Walter would hurt her. While she was outside, Walter cut himself with the broken glass. Mom decided she just couldn't handle Walter anymore, so he was sent to live at the regional facility for children with mental retardation.

The staff at the regional facility ran "behavior management" programs on Walter. They pinned him to the floor in "personal restraint" when he was aggressive or started destroying property. They put him in isolation time-out, but he got so agitated that he hit his head against the walls until his ears were puffed up like a prizefighter's. One afternoon, in a fit of rage, Walter broke all the windows in the sheltered workshop building. The staff decided he was "crazy" and had him transferred to the nearby state psychiatric hospital.

Walter was placed in the psychiatric hospital's rehabilitation unit because of his developmental disability. He was a large young man by this time, and still very angry. He stole food and personal items from the other people who lived on his ward. In his frequent tantrums he bit people, sometimes seriously. After many biting incidents, the medical staff took a desperate measure. They pulled all of his teeth! Walter could no longer bite people, but he didn't like the pureed food he had to eat. That made him mad. He learned to poke people in the eye.

When I met Walter it was because the organization I worked for at the time was going to help him move out of the psychiatric hospital and into a six-bed group home in a nearby small town. There were many planning sessions leading up to Walter's move. Most of the sessions revolved around deciding how we were going to deal with Walter's aggressive behavior.

I was fortunate at the time to be working with a psychologist who had a deeper understanding of people with disabilities than the usual kneejerk application of behavioral principles. I'll call him "Dr. Mac." Dr. Mac knew that reinforcers work better than punishers, but he also knew Walter was probably going to try his old behavior in the new situation. We were, therefore, going to have to keep Walter from hurting his housemates and breaking up the house, while at the same time showing Walter a better way to get what he needed.

Dr. Mac helped us set up a program whereby if Walter attacked someone (usually eye poking), he would be moved quickly to the living room and held in a chair until he settled down. That may sound like the old "restraint and time-out" routine that hadn't worked in his previous placements. But there were some critical differences. The sitting in the chair in the living room was only a protective intervention, to keep Walter from hurting people. We didn't figure being held in a chair was going to "teach Walter a lesson," we just wanted to keep people from being hurt.

The lesson came with the positive part of the program. As we got to know Walter, we came to understand that he liked attention from staff and he liked coffee. Though Walter only used a few words of spoken language, he seemed to have a pretty good idea of what people were communicating to him. When he first arrived at the group home, I sat down with him and said, "Walter, I think you're going to like your new home here. But it's not like the hospital. We want you to be happy and have what you want. But we can't let you hurt other people." I then explained the reason for the living room chair restraint. I continued, "If you can get ready to go to work in the morning and not try to hurt anybody, someone will sit down with you here in the dining room and you can have another cup of coffee." He understood that part. "Coffee, coffee, coffee," he said, with a big toothless grin.

Now wouldn't this be a delightful fairy tale, if that's all it took, if after 20 years of harsh institutional treatment I told Walter to "be good" and he said, "Sure, James; I'll get right on it." Of course, that's not how it happened. Some mornings, Walter tried to poke the eyes of his more vulnerable housemates. Two staff had to wrestle him to the living room chair. He broke his bedroom window once. He got hold of some matches at the workshop and returned home to start a small fire on his bedroom chair. The first month Walter lived in the group home, we recorded 95 episodes of aggression or property damage. (Remember data collection?) Several staff quit in fear of Walter's outbursts.

There were also mornings when Walter was a pleasant, even humorous companion. Staff would joke with him, and his laugh put everyone in a good mood. On such mornings staff were vocal in their praise of Walter. "Walter, you are doing great this morning. You haven't bothered anybody and you're ready to go to work. Since you've been being good, let's sit down and have another cup of coffee." Walter would grin and say, "Be good, be good, be good. Coffee, coffee, coffee."

The second month, Walter's aggressive episodes dropped to 40. Even these were not so intense, more testing of the limits than full-scale attacks. Some of the staff took a real liking to the Walter who was coming out— a funny, affectionate guy who liked attention and was very helpful to people who treated him with respect.

The third month, Walter's aggression was very infrequent and of low intensity. Staff began to be able to recognize when Walter was starting to get upset. They learned how to help him calm down by getting him involved in a different activity (redirection).

In three months, Walter had gone from being the toothless terror of the rehabilitation ward to being just a simple guy who liked to go to the mall and keep his room clean. What happened? Did his disability go away? Was he cured? This chapter looks at how to deal effectively with challenges like those Walter presented.

"BAD" BEHAVIOR

When I started working at Colin Anderson Center, I saw lots of "bad" behavior. There were screaming tantrums and fights and broken furniture. One guy in Boys Cottage constantly punched himself in the face until his eyes were puffed shut. A woman in the ECHO Deaf-Blind unit hit her forehead on the floor when she was upset. One night she hit it so hard, she detached the retina in her eye.

Some of the strange behaviors had names. "Ruminating" was bringing food back up from the stomach and chewing it again. "Pica" was eating things that weren't food (t-shirts, magic markers, paper). I had never seen such behavior, and I figured these strange people must act that way because they had mental retardation. I thought wild behavior was part of the disability. I never asked myself the deeper question: Do people act the way they do because they have mental retardation or because of the way they have been treated (because they have mental retardation)?

As for what to do about "bad" behavior, one old time ward aide named Junior gave me a powerful lesson on my first day on Big Boys ward. Junior asked me if I had had "that behavior management crap" in my training. I told him I had. He said, "Let me tell you what's really going on here." He pointed to a large man named George, a man who intimidated by his very look. "You see George over there? If George gets out of hand, I just get right up to him and let him have it between the eyes." Junior smacked his fist loudly into his palm for effect. "'Cause if I don't, I might as well give George my keys and go home."

Junior was serious. He truly believed his job was to control the men who lived in that ward. The way Junior saw it, they were retarded and he was the staff. It was as if he was the Boss and they were the inmates. There was no attempt to understand who the men were or why they acted the way they did. There was nothing but a power struggle. And since Junior had the keys, the strait jackets, and the nurse with a hypodermic needle, he felt like he could always win the struggle.

The problem as I saw it was that the struggle was never ending.

"CHALLENGING" BEHAVIOR

Instead of calling these troublesome behaviors "bad" I think it's better to refer to them as "challenging" behavior. Why do we call it that? Who does this behavior challenge? Well, it's certainly a challenge to those of us who deal with it day after day in our work. No one likes to be cursed or spit at or punched.

I'd like you to consider, though, that this kind of behavior is even more of a challenge to the people who act that way. In many people with disabilities, their behavior, the way they act when they're frustrated or unhappy or angry, is much more of an obstacle to their success than is their inability to read or speak or walk. Most people will be very understanding and helpful when they see that a person has difficulty doing things. They will not be so understanding when they see people acting in ways that are unacceptable in civilized society.

Understanding that a person's behavior is an obstacle to his success leads to an understanding that in trying to change that behavior you are not trying to control the person. Rather, you are trying to help him control himself...and thereby be more successful.

"...TO GET WHAT THEY WANT."

So why do people act the way they do? The simplest answer is that "People do what they do to get what they want." This is just another way of saying people do certain behaviors in order to get reinforcers. This is a simplified way of looking at things, but think about it regarding your own behavior. Don't you act in ways that will get you the things, relationships and events you would like in your life? And don't you try to avoid doing the things that will make bad things happen or make people think badly of you? This part of the answer of why people act the way they do is universal. It has nothing to do with whether a person has a disability. But there's more.

People also act on their beliefs. We do the things we believe will get us what we want. If our beliefs are a true reflection of what happens in the world, our actions will be successful. If, on the other hand, our beliefs are mistaken, we will act in ways that don't get us what we want. And we won't understand why our behavior isn't working the way we'd like it to.

Imagine, then, that you're a person who has trouble understanding the connections between behavior and consequences. The world goes by pretty fast for you, and you can't seem to figure out how to work it. Even as a child, you were frustrated because Mom expected you to be able to do things (like pee in the potty) that you just never learned the how or why of. As an adult, you don't follow language very well and can't keep up with the social by-play that is the way to win friends and influence people.

You can learn, however. As you get bigger, you learn to use threats and intimidation to run an extortion racket. You howl and bite and people stop trying to make you do things you don't want to do. You scream and break things and people pay attention to you. You push your little brother off his chair and get some extra food from the dinner table. You do what you do because it works.

In the institutional environment, where attention is hard to get, you learn to curse loudly, to injure yourself, to defecate in your pants—these things always get attention. If you want to be somebody (and who doesn't?), you push your weight around. You can be the one who is feared, the baddest badass on the ward. This kind of behavior is sometimes called "maladaptive," because it is a bad ("mal") way to get along ("adapt") in the world. But is it really? Isn't it really adaptive in the world in which you live? It works, in a way. So why change it?

We are sneaking up on an understanding of the first lesson in dealing with challenging behavior: People do what they do because it works; it's "functional." Being aware of this gives us the basic secret of behavioral change: Set up a situation where the old behavior no longer works (functions), but be sure to replace it with a new way for the person to get what she wants.

That's what happened with Walter. We shut down the aggression he had used as a way of asserting himself, of having his own way and being somebody. It no longer worked. Then we helped him learn to replace that old way of acting with a new way that got him even more of what he wanted. The new way works even better, because it works in the community at large. Walter's improved behavior brought him more freedom, more friends, and more self satisfaction. It was hard work to get him to see where he might go if he cleaned up his act. But when he finally did, there was great reward not only for Walter, but also for the staff (who also preferred an extra cup of coffee in the morning to holding Walter in a chair). When behavior improves, everybody wins.

HOW DOES THIS BEHAVIOR WORK?

Some functions of behavior:
- Get attention
- Give information
- Avoid an activity or task
- Express feelings
- Get stimulation or physical contact
- Get permission
- Ask for assistance

Many times I have heard reports like "George jumped up and started hitting me for no reason." Usually, as I looked deeper into the situation, I discovered plenty of reasons. The only times I've seen a person act "with no reason" is when he was suffering from hallucinations or delusions of mental illness. In those cases, the "reasons" were all inside him, part of the thing that was torturing his mind. For all other behavior, there was a reason. When you support a person with disabilities who has challenging behaviors, your first job is to figure out "why."

You are going to have to understand how the behavior in question functions (works) for the person who is doing it. What is the behavior meant to accomplish?

If you have taken the time and attention to develop a relationship with the person you support, you will know a lot about what she wants. Her behavior will have communicated her desires and preferences, what she wants out of life. Once you get this piece of the puzzle, you are well on your way to being able to help her change her behavior to something that is more acceptable to her family, friends, neighbors and co-workers.

The notion of "listening" to behavior may seem strange to you. We're used to listening to what people say with their words. But some people don't use words for communication. Can you imagine how frustrating it must be not to be able to communicate even the fact that you have a headache and want to be left alone? Then imagine how helpful it would be if someone took the time to figure out what was bothering you. When we pay close attention to what the person is communicating to us, we can often reduce the frequency (how often) and intensity (how strong) of behavioral outbursts just by helping him get what he needs.

When Ricky moved to the new group home from the state facility, he had a very bad reputation. When agitated or frustrated, Ricky would bite his hand and jump up and down, yelling and moaning. People had tried to restrain him to make him stop, but he had used his 220 pounds to hurt them. We decided we were going to do things differently.

Ricky's new program was: When Ricky gets agitated, stay with him and encourage him to show you what's bothering him. No restraint, no punishment—just understanding and attention.

I remember one evening watching Ricky get very frustrated about something and start into his usual jumping and moaning. A young woman who worked in Ricky's home, a person half his size, gently held his hands while he jumped. She looked him in the eye and said, "Show me what's wrong, Ricky." She wasn't afraid of him. She wasn't trying to control him. It was great.

Ricky finally took the young woman into the living room and showed her that the headphones for his stereo had broken. She helped him put the headphones back together. But more importantly, she began the process of showing Ricky he did not have to get agitated in order to be heard.

Sometimes it's hard to figure out how a behavior works. The person is usually not going to come up to you and say "I smack Nora because it makes the staff come running. Then they put their hands all over me, and I like the contact." It will probably take close observation and data collection and analysis by an experienced team. But the answer is always there.

Sometimes it helps to start with yourself. When asking why she acts that way, we have to ask ourselves why we act the way we do. Why do we do things that don't make sense? Why do we do things that don't get us what we want, that drive people away, that cause us to fail in our attempts at having a life?

One possible reason is that we have been formed by our experience to act a certain way. Consider the experience of a person with mental retardation who has had difficulty understanding what is going on and whose behavior has caused people to become frustrated, impatient and possibly abusive with her. Can we not get some understanding of why she acts the way she does?

Add to the experience of having a mind that processes things with difficulty the almost universal institutional experience of abandonment, neglect and outright abuse, and it should not be surprising that you encounter a person who is feisty, angry, and aggressive. Wouldn't you be?

OBSERVING BEHAVIOR

Consider yourself a behavioral Private Investigator. Your job is to track down the clues that will lead you to understand the function of the behavior that is an obstacle to the person you support. Your investigation will require close observation and shrewd thinking. You can do it, but don't neglect to ask for guidance from your more experienced colleagues and from the trained professionals on your team. It may take everyone's best ideas to come up with the best solution.

You may be asked to record data about when and how things happen. It is very important that you observe closely and record accurately. Looking at patterns of behavior over weeks or even months is sometimes the only way to see what's going on. And knowing what's going on is the only way to intervene successfully. Your observations may be the key to the puzzle.

MULTI-MODAL INVESTIGATION

Remember our old friends Antecedent, Behavior, and Consequence? I hope you remember that Antecedent is the thing that comes before the Behavior and causes it to happen. Well, that would be a handy thing to know when you're dealing with a challenging behavior, wouldn't it? What was the Antecedent? What set this off? What made this behavior occur right now and not earlier in the day? Did something happen to the person to cause him to act this way?

Dr. William Gardner is an experienced behavioral sleuth. He has developed a method he calls "Multi-Modal." That's just a big university term for looking at the thing from a lot of different perspectives.

Dr. Gardner has taught us that when it comes to challenging behavior, there are a number of different ways to look at Antecedents. He calls these different perspectives Vulnerability, Setting, and Trigger. They are like the detective's magnifying glass, helping us to look more closely at the kinds of things that might lead to a behavioral outburst.

VULNERABILITY

The first of Dr. Gardner's tools is Vulnerability. A Vulnerability is something about the person that makes them more likely to act in a certain way. A Vulnerability could be something from the person's past that makes today's situation scary or stressful to them. For example, I once worked with a woman who would take a bath but would pitch a tantrum if asked to take a shower. She didn't use words, so she couldn't explain her resistance. But one of the staff who had worked with her years before reported that at the state psychiatric facility the woman had been given cold showers as punishment for toileting accidents. Why does she act that way? Because something from her past (a Vulnerability) has made her afraid of the current situation.

A Vulnerability could also be something about how the person thinks, something to do with the nature of their disability. It's hard for anyone to make changes in the way he acts, but it's even harder for people who have difficulty learning stuff or understanding what's going on or who may have damage to the part of their brains that controls a particular kind of behavior.

Edward, for example, was a man who had tantrums some days when he came home from the workshop and found that his mother was not there to visit him. He would yell and cry and tear up his bed, despite the fact that we tried to explain to him that his mother would come on Friday and today was only Wednesday. The problem was that Edward didn't understand the days of the week. That was a Vulnerability, something about him that made him likely to get upset because he didn't understand what was going on.

In Edward's case, our being aware of this Vulnerability led directly to a solution. We put a large calendar on his bedroom wall. On the squares for Fridays, we put a picture of his mother. Each day when Edward came home from work, he X'd out that day and excitedly pointed to how many days were left before Mom came to see him.

SETTING

The next tool in the Multi-Modal bag of tricks is called Setting. The Setting is the time and place and circumstances when the challenging behavior is likely to occur. Think of setting as cocking the hammer of the gun. It doesn't make the behavior occur (that's Trigger, the next tool); but it means the conditions are ripe.

When you're looking at the Setting, you have to observe and record things about the behavior. What time of day did it occur? What day of the week? Who was present when the behavior started? Is there a particular person who seems to agitate the person you're observing? Is the behavior more likely to occur in crowded, noisy places or at quiet times when the person may be expressing boredom?

Sometimes, especially for people who can't talk, medical issues can serve as Settings. The person may be in pain, or constipated, or hungry and not understand why he is feeling so bad. All kinds of things can serve as Settings for a behavioral outburst.

TRIGGER

Settings don't cause challenging behaviors; they just set up ripe conditions for them. The immediate cause, the thing that happens just before the behavior, is called a Trigger. It could be a word, a touch, a noise, a request. Bam! When the Trigger is pulled, behavior can go from zero to sixty in a heartbeat. Suddenly the person you were working with is yelling, slapping herself, hitting at you, throwing things. When large adults throw tantrums it is a scary and awesome sight for all involved. Why, then, is it important to know what Triggers a behavior? So you can avoid pulling the Trigger!

I have worked with people who thought their job was to control the behavior of the people they were "in charge of." They paid no attention to what caused a behavior to happen, figuring instead that they could control the behavior by applying Consequences (usually punishers) after it happened. I've seen staff willfully trigger a behavioral outburst in an obviously agitated person, because the staff knew that once the person started to tantrum he could be put into restraint or seclusion and the staff person wouldn't have to deal with him anymore. The staff's attitude was "He needs to learn what happens when he acts that way." That kind of staff behavior is not professional; it is abusive.

When you develop your skills of observation and analysis, you will learn to understand people's Vulnerabilities. You will help the people you work with avoid stressful Settings and obvious Triggers. This is called changing the environment rather than the person. It is a very respectful and sophisticated way to work. You will have more fun, develop better relationships and be seen as more successful, if you work to understand a person's behavior rather than merely controlling it for him. People will begin to remark, "She's so good with him. He never acts that way when he's with her."

WORKING WITH CONSEQUENCES

So far we've just been talking about how to work with Antecedents, what happens before the challenging behavior. But we can also affect behavior by using what comes after, the Consequences of the behavior.

"If you don't behave, you'll suffer the consequences," your father said. You knew he was talking about punishment— "If you do something bad, something bad will happen to you." You would have to go to your room, lose a privilege, be grounded, or maybe even endure a spanking. Do you remember those times? How did they make you feel? Did the punishment fill you with a burning desire to always be good? Or did it maybe make you think about not getting caught next time? Did it make you feel closer to the person punishing you, or did you secretly wish to get even? Did the punishment teach you a better way to act?

Remember the behaviorist's definition of a Punisher: It's something the person doesn't like and will work to avoid. And if it follows a Behavior, the Behavior will be less likely to occur again. It sure worked for the pigeon, didn't it? The researchers shocked his feet every time he pecked the lever...and he quickly stopped the Behavior.

Here's where I reveal another of my biases. I've used Punishers a lot over the years of my human service career. I've held people face down on the floor ("prone restraint"), strapped them into a special chair with

Velcro straps, sprayed cold water and lemon juice in their faces, shocked them with little cattle prods ("shock boxes"), locked them in closets ("isolation time-out"), tied them up in "sleeves" (strait jackets), and taken away all manner of privileges (smoke breaks, home visits, vacations, desserts).

And you know what? None of it ever made a person's behavior improve.

Our punishers did not work in real life the way they did in theories that had been developed from animal experiments. When this happened, the failure was usually blamed on the staff. They must not have been running the program right.

With apologies to all the behavioral psychologists who have been my friends, my allies and my teachers, I call the years we did all those terrible things to people the "reign of behavioral terrorism." I'm glad it's mostly over now. Most provider agencies and state regulatory bodies now prohibit the kinds of things we did in the name of "scientific behaviorism."

The fact that punishment gets out of hand and tends to become abuse is good enough reason to stay away from using it. But there's an even stronger reason—it just doesn't work.

GARDNER'S LAW

Here's where I have to introduce you to what I call "Gardner's Law." It comes from the same Dr. Bill Gardner who gave us Multi-Modal behavior analysis. Dr. Gardner is a professor of behavioral psychology, but he's also a practical man, a Mississippi gentleman. One afternoon, just a few years ago, a high powered group of psychologists, social workers and other assorted professional types was gathered in a conference room at a large state mental retardation facility. We had asked Dr. Gardner to consult with us about a young man who was supposed to move out of the facility into a community-based home.

The problem was that the man was "on a program" that required staff to put wrist and leg shackles on him if he did an aggressive "target behavior." For two years, the man had carried his "restraint gear" around in a gym bag, and a male staff person who was trained in how to "apply" the restraints always accompanied him.

The psychologists had a long graph (several pieces of paper taped together) detailing the man's rate of aggression for the past two years. Dr. Gardner studied the graph while the professionals sat hushed like a bunch of eager graduate students. Then he looked up from the paper and said, "What I can tell from this graph is that sometimes this behavior happens more and sometimes it happens less. There's no evidence that this restraint program has done what it's supposed to do." Then he uttered those profound words, the words of someone deeply committed to making a real difference in people's lives: "The way I see it, *If you're doing something and it doesn't work, you ought to stop doing that and do something else.*" I started to think of this as Gardner's Law.

It doesn't seem so profound on the surface, does it? It just seems like common sense. When you do something that is supposed to change someone's behavior in a way that will make his life better, you ought to have a way of measuring whether it does that or not. And if it doesn't work, especially if it's something obnoxious like leg shackles, then you better stop doing it.

Let me repeat what I said above. In over twenty years, I have never, not once, seen a situation in which punishers made a person's behavior improve. Punishers are clearly something that doesn't work. So we ought to stop using them and try something different.

THE CARROT AND THE STICK

The "something different" can best be illustrated by the story of the carrot and the stick. Suppose I am driving a donkey cart, and I want to go into town. I smack the donkey on the rump with a long stick to make him go. What does he do? He kicks at the cart and lays down. The harder I hit him, the louder he refuses. But I've got a better idea. I know that this donkey likes carrots. So I tie a bunch of carrots to the end of the stick and dangle them in front of his nose. Up gets the donkey and trots off in pursuit of those tasty carrots. I'm headed for town...and the donkey will enjoy a luscious carrot feast. Everybody wins.

SETTING LIMITS

Before we go on to how to use carrots rather than sticks, let me be clear about one thing. My proposal to get rid of punishers doesn't mean that the people we work with can "get away with murder" or "do anything they want." We do have to set limits. We cannot allow people to seriously hurt themselves or others. We cannot allow them to threaten or exploit others. But setting limits is very different from applying punishers.

When we set clear limits, we say, "This far and no further." Sometimes this involves our physically getting in someone's way, blocking a punch, or holding his hands down. There are different techniques for these protective interventions, and you should be trained in one of the systems that allows you to fearlessly stand your ground. But standing your ground and saying, "I'm not going to let you hurt me" is very different from saying, "If you hit me, I'll take away your privileges."

Setting limits is not doing something to the people you support. Rather, it can be a way of building a protective fence around them, within which they can behave successfully. Just as crutches might keep someone from falling, a support person who can firmly but respectfully set limits can help keep a person from falling into old behavioral habits.

People who have been managed using punishment, will often do what is called "limit testing." They'll push and poke to see how far they can go before you lower the boom on them. If you're not going to lower the boom, you'd better stand your ground. Be willing to show the person clearly where the limits are and that you cannot be moved. If you pass the test, the person will probably not feel the need to keep testing. If you waiver, the person will keep on pushing to see how much he can flex the limits. (This works with teenagers, too.)

TIME-OUT'S FULL NAME

One way to set limits is through the intelligent use of "time-out." I said "intelligent" use, because in the past we have called a lot of things "time-out" that were really just punishers in disguise. We would lock a person in a closet and call it "isolation time-out." Or we would take away a person's right to go outside and call it "time-out."

We did these things because we forgot time-out's full name, which is "time-out from reinforcers." Time-out from reinforcers means that as long as you are acting a certain way, good things (reinforcers) are happening for you. When you get off the path and start acting in a "bad" way, the reinforcers stop flowing. We don't take anything away from you. We don't do something to you that you don't like. We just turn off the reinforcer faucet until you start acting the way that gets reinforcers.

Think of this as either facing the person you are working with or turning your back to him. When the person is acting in a way that is respectful of others and leads to successes in his life, you are right there with him. You tell him he's a great guy…and you mean it. You do fun and rewarding things with him. But if he steps off the path, everything comes to a halt. "No good things come when you talk to me that way." But, and here's where time-out is different from punishment, as soon as you get back on the track, those carrots are back, enriching your life.

Using the signal of being "in" the reinforcer flow or "out" of it is sort of like the instrument guidance system a small airplane would use. Wander off the flight path and an electronic tone warns you you are off and need to make a correction. When you use time-out appropriately you become a sort of "artificial conscience" for the person you're working with, guiding him in the direction of success and satisfaction.

Just as a child keeps an eye on Mom for clues on how he's behaving, the person you support may keep an eye on you for encouraging smiles or discouraging scowls. Even subtle body language cues and tone of voice serve as powerful guides to the person who doesn't use spoken language. If your cues lead the person to successfully getting what she wants and needs, she will look to you often. You will then develop the reputation of being someone who "she really responds to."

Another advantage to using the carrots technique is that it constantly gives the person you're guiding the chance to be rewarded for doing the right thing. That doesn't always happen when you use punishers. Sometimes punishers just keep escalating until the person being punished has nothing left. Then, as Bob Dylan said, "When you ain't got nothin', you've got nothin' to lose." That's when all hell breaks loose. A person who's got nothing left to lose is a very dangerous person who doesn't care anymore about consequences.

NATURAL CONSEQUENCES

You may recall the idea of "generalization" from Chapter 7. We said new skills should be taught in the environment in which they are going to be practiced. That way, a person won't have to "generalize" their behavior from one situation to another.

Dealing with challenging behaviors should have the same concern. But there are still a lot of motivational programs that reward people with points or poker chips that can be "cashed in" on various prizes and privileges. The problem with this is that no one uses points or poker chips in the real world. How are you going to learn to act right in the neighborhood if you're used to working for poker chips?

Better than the artificial rewards that sometimes come with written behavior intervention plans, is the use of "natural consequences." Natural consequences are exactly what they sound like—the thing that naturally happens after you do a certain behavior.

Natural consequences can be both negative and positive. People with disabilities have often been excluded from the positive consequences of being a good neighbor, a valued co-worker, or a cherished lover. But they have also been protected from natural consequences of the painful kind. We don't want to see them embarrassed or fired or shunned, so we make excuses for their behavior and let them off the hook. They don't learn to act any better. Which means they are eventually segregated and shunned anyway.

Sometimes protecting people with disabilities from natural consequences is actually a put down, a sign that we don't respect them enough to let them learn from their own experience and their own mistakes. Often, if we just get out of their way, they figure it out from the reaction they get in the real world. I once asked Bobby why he acted so well on his job but then got into aggressive power struggles with his group home staff on the weekends. He looked at me like I was stupid. "If I acted that way at work, I'd get fired." Natural consequences.

People who have learned how to fight the system are amazed by natural consequences. Larry had a part-time job, so he went to one of those rent-to-own places and got a stereo system for his room. One day at work he decided he'd had enough and loudly walked off the job. Come Friday, he didn't get paid. Come Saturday, the repo man was at Larry's door to collect either that week's payment or the stereo. Larry had to give up his system. You don't argue with the repo man the way you argue with your group home staff. Come Monday, Larry was looking for another job.

One day Willie came up to me, very excited, and said, "Guess what, James. I've got my own cable service now." I told him that was great, that he must feel good that he kept his job and had money to spend. "Yeah," he continued, "and you know what? If I don't pay my cable bill, they cut off my cable." Natural consequences. Welcome to the real world, Willie.

PERSON-CENTERED BEHAVIOR STRATEGIES

If you work with anyone who has challenging behaviors, you are bound to run into a "behavior management plan" or "behavior support plan." (Using the word "support" is supposed to make the plan less intrusive. It is often just window dressing.) These plans are usually written by a licensed psychologist or other behavioral specialist. If the plan requires the use of restrictive procedures (punishers) it probably has to have the written permission of the person it's written for (or their guardian) and the approval of some sort of human rights oversight committee or peer review board.

Behavior management plans usually start with a little background information about the person the plan is for, followed by a history of less restrictive interventions that were tried and failed. Then the plan tells you what the "target behavior" is. That's the behavior you want to see less of. Then there's the "intervention"—what you're supposed to do whenever the target behavior happens. Last, there is a documentation plan—what kind of record you need to keep of each occurrence of the target behavior. The person who wrote the plan will collect the documentation (data) at some interval, in order to see whether the plan is having the desired result.

I've worked in group homes (as the behaviorist) where every person who lived there had the kind of management plan described above. Everybody had target behaviors. Everybody had interventions. Everybody had data sheets. All staff had to be trained on how to implement the plans. It all seemed very scientific and orderly.

Once again, we have to apply Our Standard—"Is this the kind of life I would like to live?" Would you like to be "put on a program?" Would you like people coming into your home who are trained to implement interventions when you do a target behavior? Me neither.

What we end up with, more often than not, is a power struggle. We run our interventions on people, and they try to sabotage the program. There is one simple rule for power struggles—when you engage in a power struggle, everybody loses. The person you are trying to control loses his freedom and the understanding of how to be a responsible adult. You lose a relationship of equality with him and the opportunity to use your best heart skills in helping him learn what he needs to know to be successful. Everyone is trapped.

There is a way out. Let's call it "person-centered behavior strategies." It's person-centered because the person who needs to learn a new way to act is the center of the process. We find out from him how he wants to be supported at times when he is struggling with his behavior. And these are "strategies" rather than "plans" because they are not written in stone. They're flexible ways of dealing with behavioral challenges as they come up, allowing you to use your common sense, your intuition, and your relationship with the person you support.

COMMUNICATION LEADS TO UNDERSTANDING

You begin developing a person-centered behavior strategy by communicating with the person whose behavior is seen as challenging. I say "communicate," rather than "talk," because you will sometimes be working with people who don't use words for their communication.

What do you communicate about? Well, the first thing you want to know is what is the function or purpose of the behavior you'd like to change. We talked about that earlier. Once you have some idea how that behavior works for that person, you'll know what she thinks she is getting through doing it. Don't be fooled, though. Many people with developmental disabilities don't have good "insight." That is, they don't have a good understanding of what it is they really want. That's not to say we should decide for them. It's just that they may need help understanding what's available in life and what motivates them to act the way they do. Don't you?

While you're communicating about the function of behavior, don't forget the possibility that some behavior is a symptom of an underlying mental or physical illness. Ronald, for example, started episodes of screaming and hitting himself in the side of the head. He couldn't describe what was happening. His behavior was our only clue. We took him to the doctor for examination and discovered he had a severe ear infection. Because Ronald didn't understand about infections, he was hitting at the thing that hurt him, trying to make it go away.

When his infection was treated, he stopped hitting himself. We never could have changed his behavior through strategies of reward and motivation.

Be careful, too, about behaviors that might be symptoms of underlying mental illness. Mental illness can change a person's whole motivation structure.

In psychotic disorders, the person sometimes reacts to things that are going on inside his head (delusions, hallucinations) more than to what we're doing to help. For instance, Pat reported he heard good voices in one ear and bad voices in the other. He was very resistant to the audiologist's prescription that he ought to be wearing a hearing aid in his right ear. It was the one that heard the bad voices; and he didn't want to hear them any more clearly.

In affective (mood) disorders, a person can be literally incapable of doing what's good for her. Depression, for instance, can make it hard to even get out of bed. Nothing is enjoyable, and people seem distant and judgmental. Manic episodes can cause a person to stop sleeping, spend all their money, and become edgy and paranoid.

If a person has mental health needs, those needs must be dealt with through the appropriate treatment before any kind of behavioral strategies have a chance of being effective.

TURNING THINGS AROUND

Once you figure out what the behavior is really trying to get, what the person really wants, you need to find some strategies that will work to turn things around. You want to close off one way of acting, while opening up a new way, all the while paying close attention to the desires and tolerance of the person you're working with. It's a big job. You may need help from other team members. But never lose sight of who these strategies are serving. And never forget Our Standard.

The first place to turn when looking for strategies is the person who is experiencing the behavioral challenge. If she can communicate with you, ask her, "What do you think we should do to help you change this behavior?" If she says, "I'm not going to change and you can't make me," your first step will be to help her understand what carrots will be available to her if she makes the change. You have to do that first, because you can't force anyone do the right thing. Unless she sees value in the change, she will fight you every step of the way. That's why it's so important the strategies be person-centered.

Maybe she won't resist the change. Maybe she already knows her behavior pushes people away and got her fired from her last job. She may have a suggestion that could work. It will be tailored to address her specific challenges and make use of her personal abilities. And, best of all, she will be invested in it. This is the best way to go.

TOOLS YOU CAN USE

What if the person you're working with can come up with nothing helpful? What if you have to come up with strategies on your own?

There are a few tips I can give you. Think of them as tools for helping people deal with challenging behavior.

IGNORE AND REDIRECT

The first tool is the one that will be most useful, day in and day out. It is simply to ignore behaviors that are more an annoyance than a real challenge. I have a little rule that will be helpful: "Ignore what you can."

Many times challenging behaviors are old attention getters, learned long ago and no longer useful. In that case, the less attention you pay the behavior the better. Just act like it didn't happen and move on to something else.

Be clear that I didn't tell you to ignore the person...just the behavior. If the person is cursing to get your attention and you ignore him by refusing to interact with him at all, what do you think he's likely to do? That's right—curse even more. He's looking for attention, remember. You need to give him some attention. Just act like the attention is the usual kind that you give all the time because you care about him, not brought about by the cursing. The lesson needs to be that he doesn't need to curse to get your attention. In fact, you're going to pay no attention at all to cursing.

You can see how well this strategy works when you see what happens to someone who doesn't use it. One day, the training coordinator at the sheltered workshop called me about Bart. She said he had been going up to female staff and grabbing their breasts. Most of the women who worked there were pretty savvy about this kind of thing, so they just lightly brushed his hands aside and asked him which job he was supposed to be working at. One young woman, though, freaked out every time he did it. She would turn red, grab Bart's hands and yell into his face, "Bart, you stop that! You know how much that upsets me." Well, Bart did indeed know how much it upset her. That's why he started targeting her. Touching the breasts was not the reinforcer for Bart; the attention he got for touching the breasts was.

Remember that lack of attention is one of the main characteristics of the institutional mindset. The person who goes quietly about his business is ignored, while the one who raises a ruckus gets all the attention he needs. That means you'll see a lot of inappropriate attempts at getting attention. Ignore them and they'll go away.

But don't forget the redirect part. "Redirect" means to get the person's behavior going in another direction. Another of my behavior rules is "don't try to stop a person from doing something...get him to do something different." The young woman who tried to get Bart to stop just made the situation worse. If, instead of reacting, she had just ignored his inappropriate touching and said, "Bart, are you on break or should you be returning to your work station?" she would have redirected Bart's attention to a more appropriate concern.

When ignore and redirect are used gracefully and seamlessly, they function much like some moves in judo. Instead of confronting and struggling with the issue, you use the energy to smoothly avoid conflict. Ignore and redirect should become second nature to you. You will hardly be aware you're using a technique, but you will know your days are easier; and the person you're supporting will waste less of her (and your) time playing challenging games.

OFFER OPTIONS

The second skill in this behavioral toolkit is to always offer options. Options are choice points. Do you want A or B? When you offer options rather than stating directives, you allow a person to choose his own path, and you avoid power struggles.

Let's say it's 7:30 AM at the group home. Breakfast is over, and it's time to get everyone on the van to go to work. Mona starts her shift at the greenhouse, a job she's held for two years, at 8:00 You see that Mona is sitting sulkily in the La-Z-Boy in the living room. You don't want to have any trouble that upsets the schedule, so you bark at her, "OK, Mona; time to go to work. Get on the van. We haven't got all day." Mona, who does have all day, barks back, "NO!" You respond, "Mona, I'm not gonna go through this with you again. I can call James and we'll both put you on the van, whether you like it or not. So move." Mona digs in. "No!" she shouts. "I'm not going!" Well, now haven't we got a nice power struggle on our hands here? And what happens in a power struggle? Yep, everyone loses.

Let's rewind this tape and see if we can do it better. You approach Mona and ask gently, "Hey, Mona, is there anything you need before you leave for work?" You're centering on her and her needs, rather than the schedule. Mona says, "No, I'm not going to work." Sometimes people don't go to work because they're sick, so you ask Mona, "Are you not feeling well?" She replies, "No, I'm just not going. And you can't make me." You hear the challenge in her voice, but you ignore it. You're thinking that since she's not sick, she may just be looking to exert control over her life. You ask, "Well, you know they're counting on you at the greenhouse. They'll really miss you if you don't show up." You can see by Mona's face that's she's softening her attitude. She likes to hear that stuff about being needed. "OK," she says, "I'll go." That's a ball you can pick up and run with. You say, "Oh, that's great, Mona. You know, we only have a few minutes before it's time to go, would you like to have another quick cup of coffee, or would you like to fill the birdfeeder?" Now Mona's attitude has really changed. She's no longer thinking about how much fun it's going to be to kick your butt on the way to the van. Instead, she's thinking about which activity to choose. You have shifted the focus of the interaction from getting her to obey a command to asking what she'd like to do. She feels in control; so she doesn't need to struggle with you. "I think I'd like to fill the birdfeeder," she proclaims. "OK," you reply, "you know where the seed is. Do you need any help?" Once Mona gets rolling (out of the defensive La-Z-Boy posture) you probably won't have any trouble with her getting on the van. And you'll both have a better day.

If you've been in this situation before, you may be asking, "Yeah, but what if I give her an option and she says she doesn't want to do either thing?"

No problem. You ask, "Mona, before we go, would you like to have another quick cup of coffee, or would you like to fill the birdfeeder?" She digs in, preferring the power struggle to the chance to choose. You don't take the bait. Breezily, you say, "OK; well, you think about it and I'll check back with you in a few minutes." Ignore, redirect, and walk away. Mona doesn't get her power struggle, and she doesn't get to fill the birdfeeder, either. Do you think she might make a choice when you come back?

Just remember that there are always options, even when you're in a situation that "has to" be done. Instead of saying, "You need to clean the house," you ask, "Would you rather do the mopping or the sweeping?" Instead of saying, "You have to take your medicine," you ask, "Would you like to take it with juice or milk?" When people have options they feel respected. They have much less need to power struggle with you.

Just be sure the options are both acceptable paths. I got a call one evening from one of the children's group homes. It concerned Benjamin, a boy who had been putting up a fuss about taking a bath before bedtime. The staff person said, "I used that options thing with Benjamin tonight, but it didn't work." I asked her what happened. "Well," she said, "I asked Benjamin if he wanted to take a bath or go to bed. And he went to bed." Benjamin wasn't stupid.

We talked about what had happened, and she decided it might have been better to ask Benjamin if he wanted to take a bath or clean his room (another task he was resisting) before he went to bed. That way, regardless of which one he chose, something would have been accomplished. Remember: "Take what you can get closest to what you want."

GIVE IN EARLY AND GRACEFULLY

You can use this one if you're a parent. There are times when you just get tired of setting limits, enforcing rules, and laying down the law. You decide to cut the person you're working with (or your four-year-old) some slack. She's really not supposed to have sugar in the evening, but tonight you don't feel like resisting her desire for another piece of apple pie. You could try to hold the line until she pushes you over the edge with her whining and threats, or you could just give in early and gracefully. If you do the first, you are teaching her that she can get what she wants by pushing you to your limit—a dangerous lesson. If you choose the second, you cruise through the evening and can still work on sugar restriction another day.

Sometimes it's not you who is close to the edge, but the person you're working with. If you know the person well and are paying attention, you'll recognize the signs that things are getting ragged. It's better to loosen up now and avoid a blow-up. He can make his bed later...or not at all. He can learn to say "please" and "thank you" some other time. We all have times when we need a little understanding. People who live in institutional environments are programmed from morning till night. It won't hurt to cut them a little slack now and then. The task is rarely so important that it's worth setting yourself up as a little dictator over it.

WHEN IT'S OVER; IT'S OVER

There will always come a time when a person's behavior goes over the edge. A tantrum will flare; a punch will be thrown; harsh words will fly. As I said above, you will need to be trained on how to protect yourself and others in the event things get physical. You can't get that kind of training from this book.

What I'd like you to learn here is very important to your success in helping a person change his behavior. That is, when it hits the fan and gets ugly and scary, ride it out and keep everyone safe...then, when it's over, it's over.

Behavioral blow-ups often last only a few minutes, but a lot of damage can be done, to bodies and to feelings. As a professional, it's your job to reassure the person who has just lost control that everything is going to be alright. Let him know no permanent damage has been done. Help him clean up the mess. Then get on with what you were going to do before the episode flared up.

This is hard to do. It may feel like you are rewarding him for "being bad." You may be tempted to say, "The way you acted this morning, do you think we're going to do anything fun today?" You may want to lecture and scold and threaten the loss of privileges. None of that will have a positive effect, and it only makes you feel better for a little while.

When you let things be over, you give the person the message that there is a reason for settling down. Remember, "when you ain't got nothin', you got nothin' to lose." If you scold and punish, why should the person stop the tantrum and get his act together? He's already lost everything, including, he thinks, your respect. So why not just blow it out the rest of the day? On the other hand, if you say, "OK; it's over. Let's clean up the mess and get on with what we were doing," he gets the message that by spending the past hour raising a ruckus he was wasting his own time. By his own behavior he put himself in time-out from reinforcers. All the good things you were going to be doing came to a halt while he kicked up a fuss. If you show him that the sooner he settles down the sooner the goodies start to flow again, you have taught a powerful lesson.

Why does she act that way? There are, as you've seen, lots of reasons. If you understand those reasons, though, you will be able to spend less time dealing with challenging behavior and more time getting on with success. Isn't that why we love our work?

Chapter 10

A MATTER OF RIGHTS

A MATTER OF RIGHTS

When it comes to the matter of the rights of people with disabilities, I'd like you to use Our Standard again. You should know it by heart—"Is this the kind of life I'd like to live?" When applied to rights, it's easier to think of it as "Is this the way I would like to be treated?" That's because, as you saw in Chapter 2, people with disabilities have often been treated badly. Why? Because they have been seen as not quite human, a "menace," not worthy of the full rights and protections other citizens are entitled to.

Or people with disabilities have been seen as incompetents, people who are unable to understand or exercise their rights in any meaningful way. When we saw them this way, we thought we needed to take responsibility for their lives. In the process of taking responsibility we took away their rights.

Or we have done things to people with disabilities because we thought it was "for their own good." We didn't see what we did to them as rights violations because we called it something else.

We locked people up without trial and called it "involuntary commitment." We still do. We've used cruel and unusual forms of punishment and called them "behavior decelerators." We've taken away people's right to marry and have a family and called it "responsible family planning." We've told people they could not communicate with their family and friends because they needed to "get used to their new surroundings." We've searched people and taken their property away from them in the name of "public safety." People with disabilities have been drugged, shocked, and chained so they'd be happier and better behaved. And none of the violations I've mentioned has been against the law. All were done in the name of "treatment."

We in the United States often take our rights for granted. We learn early in school that our Declaration of Independence stated that we were endowed by our Creator with certain rights that can't be taken away from us. We learned that those rights include "life, liberty, and the pursuit of happiness." We learned about the Bill of Rights, that we have the right of free speech, free assembly with whomever we choose, freedom to practice our religion, to vote, to be free from having our property searched or taken away from us without "due process."

We also learned that some enslaved people didn't have these rights until 75 years after the Constitution was signed. And women didn't have the right to vote until 1920. Rights are often not easily gotten. Sometimes they need to be fought for—especially if you're a member of a group that is not considered equal to everyone else.

People with disabilities have been one of those groups (along with women, people of color, and people with minority religious or political views) that have been considered less equal. Fortunately, times are changing.

EQUAL RIGHTS FOR ALL

There are lots of lists that claim to be a "Bill of Rights" for people with disabilities. These lists of rights have different wording and vary somewhat on which rights are considered most important. But you don't need to memorize a bunch of lists. That's because they all have one thing in common— people who have disabilities have the same rights and protections that other people in society have.

In the U.S. and many other countries, those rights include:

EQUAL PROTECTION AND DUE PROCESS

All individuals must have access to all of the services and opportunities that other people do. This is called "equal protection of the law." The rights guaranteed to all citizens are protected by the U.S. Constitution and can be removed or limited only by a legal due process procedure.

When something happens that seems to be a violation of our rights, we are entitled to "due process." Due process means the right to be heard in court, to bring lawsuits, to have the representation of an attorney, to face our accuser and to bring witnesses on our behalf. In short, due process makes sure we get to tell our side of the story.

Article V of the U.S. Bill of Rights says that no person shall "be deprived of life, liberty, or property, without due process of law." The right to due process means you can't limit a person's rights just because you think it would be in his (or your) best interest. He has the right to be heard, to make his case, or to have someone of his choice speak for him.

If it is necessary to restrict a person's rights for any reason, due process procedures must be followed. Before a person's rights are restricted: the person must be informed that his or her rights may be restricted, why the restriction is necessary, and what he/she can do to have the rights restored.

The person must be allowed to express his or her opinion about the situation. Don't assume a person doesn't understand his rights and won't miss them. That's not the way you would want to be treated.

If rights are restricted without a person's direct consent, the organization restricting the right must ensure that there are safeguards to protect the person's interests. Rights Committees and/or the courts are responsible for providing such protection and due process. Unfortunately, some support service providers set up a rubber stamp approval process. They get all the necessary signatures on documents that restrict rights, but due process and equal protection are not really offered.

THE RIGHT TO CONTRACT FOR, OWN AND DISPOSE OF PROPERTY

Unless restricted by a court order ("adjudication of incompetence," see bottom of page 63), people with disabilities may own property (including real estate) and decide what to do with that property. They have the right to manage their own money, deciding how it will be spent. People who have trouble understanding where their money goes should have someone available to make sure they aren't taken advantage of.

The requirement in the U.S. that you can't own property and still be eligible for Medicaid benefits has caused some terrible violations of the property rights of people with disabilities. I knew a woman, Linda, who had been adjudicated incompetent while she was in a psychiatric hospital. The hospital found a "placement" for her in a group home that was paid for by Medicaid. Her guardian, a family member, signed the papers to sell a small house that had been left to Linda by her father. The sale, they said, was necessary, so Linda could get Medicaid.

After she moved to the group home, Linda kept telling people she wasn't staying long, because she had a house she was moving to. Staff tried to explain that the house was no longer hers. Linda insisted it was. After all, she had never sold it. One afternoon, a staff person took Linda to see the house. She had to be removed from the property after she started yelling at the current owners that they had stolen her house.

EQUAL EDUCATION OPPORTUNITY

Everyone in the United States has the right to a free public education. As you learned in Chapter 2, children with developmental disabilities were once kept at home because schools had no programs to meet their educational needs. Today, equal education in the U.S. is guaranteed by law (PL94-142: Education of all Handicapped Children Act of 1975 and PL102-119: Individuals with Disabilities Education Act Amendments of 1991 [IDEA]). These laws require public schools to assess a person's needs and to provide whatever assistance or accommodation is needed for them to learn as much as they can. For more on education, see Chapter 12—Disabilities Through the Lifecycle.

EQUAL EMPLOYMENT OPPORTUNITY

The Americans with Disabilities Act of 1990 (ADA) guarantees that people cannot be kept out of a job if the employer could make a "reasonable accommodation" that would allow them to do the work. That means an employer must evaluate a person's ability to do a particular job (even if supports are needed). No one can be denied a job just because an employer believes people with a certain disability can't work.

Another area of employment rights is equal pay for equal work. People with disabilities cannot be paid less money than others would be for the work they do (unless a rehabilitation facility has a special waiver from the Department of Labor). For more on employment, see Chapter 13—A Home and a Job in the Real World.

FREEDOM FROM CRUEL AND UNUSUAL PUNISHMENT

The U.S. Constitution forbids the use of "cruel and unusual punishment." Unfortunately, the men who wrote the phrase didn't include a list of what things should be considered "cruel and unusual." Courts are making those decisions every day.

I've done a lot of cruel and unusual things to people with disabilities over the years. I've shocked people, sprayed water in their face, wrestled them to the floor, and locked them in a plywood box. The experts said these things were OK. The Human Rights Committees approved. The guardians signed the papers. I didn't have the confidence to question them. In your work, I suggest again you use Our Standard. If it seems cruel to you, question it. If it's something you've never seen before (unusual), question it.

FREEDOM OF SPEECH AND EXPRESSION

People with disabilities have the right of free speech...even if what they say makes you uncomfortable. Self-Advocacy groups support developmentally disabled individuals to speak up for themselves (see Chapter 11—Nothing About Us Without Us). That makes a lot of people uneasy. One self-advocacy publication makes it very clear what it is about. It's called, simply, "Mouth." You don't have to shut your mouth just because you have a disability and need supports.

Freedom of expression includes sexual expression. Unless restricted by a court of law, people with disabilities must be permitted the full range of sexual expression enjoyed by others. More about that in the next chapter.

THE RIGHT TO VOTE

The U.S. Constitution guarantees all Americans the right to vote and have a voice in the affairs of our country. This is an important right of citizenship, and its denial is a serious reduction in rights

Sometimes people who have been involuntarily committed to a hospital or who have been adjudicated incompetent lose their right to vote. But no state can take away a person's right to vote just because they have a disability. Check your local laws. If there is no legal barrier, you can support people's rights by helping them register to vote.

FREEDOM OF RELIGIOUS EXPRESSION

All citizens are free to choose to express any particular belief or to attend any church or religious service. People with disabilities should be assisted to practice a familiar faith or to learn about the various kinds of religious beliefs from which they can choose, if they wish.

This also means people must be free from having someone's religion imposed on them. Your faith may be the source of great power and satisfaction to you, but you need to be careful not to push a person you support into accepting those same beliefs.

FREEDOM OF ASSEMBLY

All Americans have the right to associate with whomever they please. People with disabilities have the right to have visitors, make phone calls, and have friends of their choosing.

These are just some of the rights guaranteed to all citizens. None of these rights is lost just because a person has difficulty understanding them. People with disabilities may need help and support to be sure these rights are upheld. Such assistance is called "advocacy." When you help people exercise their rights, you are an "advocate." Advocacy is a very honorable and satisfying thing to do.

ONE ADDITIONAL RIGHT

We've established that people with disabilities have the same rights as any other citizen. But that's not exactly true. People with disabilities actually have an additional right. That is the right to "appropriate treatment" in "the least restrictive setting." This right to treatment is guaranteed in the U.S. by the Developmental Disabilities Assistance and Bill of Rights Act.

Though the right to appropriate treatment is written in the law, it's not exactly clear what it means. For instance, just what is "appropriate treatment?" Who decides what's appropriate? And which setting is "least restrictive?" Does that mean the place that is freest for a person with a particular kind of disability? Or is it the place that has the least restrictions that particular person can tolerate? Or is it whatever is available in that community? Who decides?

> **SEC. 110**
> **Rights Of Individuals With Developmental Disabilities**
>
> Congress makes the following findings respecting the rights of individuals with developmental disabilities:
>
> (1) Individuals with developmental disabilities have a right to appropriate treatment, services, and habilitation for such disabilities.
>
> (2) The treatment, services, and habilitation for an individual with developmental disabilities should be designed to maximize the developmental potential of the individual and should be provided in the setting that is least restrictive of the individual's personal liberty.
>
> — Developmental Disabilities Assistance and Bill of Rights Act, 1988

The legal issues are being fought in courts everywhere. What you need to know is that there is growing legal basis for people with disabilities to be in control of their own lives. This is the legal standing behind the growing self-advocacy movement. Many people have used the law to bring about increases in freedom and dignity.

We mentioned the Olmstead Decision in Chapter 2. That's where the US Supreme Court said two women could not be kept in a large state facility against their will and desire. But there's more to be decided. The Court left open the possibility that states can use the argument that limited resources (not enough money for everyone to receive adequate community supports) means not everyone who wants to can get out of the large facilities. Stay tuned.

PROTECTION

People with developmental disabilities can be very vulnerable. They often don't understand that they have rights. If they don't use words for communication, they can't tell someone when something bad has happened to them. Even if they do speak, their stories are sometimes garbled or confused, and an abusive or exploitative person may claim they are "crazy" to make such wild accusations.

A person who has been put on a program for "non-compliance" every time she refuses to do what staff want her to do will not understand that it's OK to say "no" to abuse.

A person who doesn't understand numbers can easily be conned out of their money and property.

A person who has limited social skills and experience and who wants to be liked may go along with someone who is sexually abusive or gets them involved in criminal activity.

And sometimes people with disabilities have been so beaten down by a system of dependency and control that they just don't care anymore. They'll go along with whatever happens to them. We call this "learned helplessness."

For all of these reasons, people with disabilities may need protection. They may need someone to watch out for their safety and help them stand up for their rights. You can be that someone.

Just be sure you don't take away some rights while you're protecting others. Remember the old Medical/Custodial model? We protected people from everything. They had no opportunity to learn from their mistakes. They were deprived of the opportunity to experience the little bruises and hurts that are part of a full life. We took away their rights in the name of safety and protection.

What you need is a balanced approach. Part of that approach may be to help people make a "risk/benefits analysis." That's just a fancy phrase for something we all do everyday. We acknowledge something is risky—driving our cars, for instance—then we see if the benefit (going where we want to go) outweighs the risk. If we see more benefit, we take the risk. If not, we figure the activity is "too risky" and we look for a different course of action.

People who have a hard time figuring things out may have a hard time weighing risks and benefits. But don't do it for them. Don't decide what you think they should be able to do and not do. Instead, do it with them. Help them work it out. Go through the decision with them step by step, looking at risks and at benefits.

Having good judgment in life is hard. All of us have experienced times when we thought we were staying safe and protecting our rights but we ended up getting hurt or taken advantage of. Good judgment can be even trickier for a person who has a hard time understanding even simple ideas and who has very little experience with real life in the real world.

If the person you're working with is unable to cope with all the kinds of decisions that go into good judgment about safety and rights, help her make up her own rules. Rules are easy to follow. If Donna has trouble knowing who she should let into her apartment, help her make a list of those people you know will treat her respectfully. Then make a rule: "Only these people come into my apartment." If she can't read a written list, help her make a notebook with people's pictures in it. By offering the support of concrete rules, you may actually expand a person's areas of freedom.

It sometimes takes a good deal of creativity to protect a person's rights without being overprotective. Think of protection as being like the "graduated guidance" we talked about in the chapter about learning—give only as much help as is needed. It's a challenge that will make your work interesting and the other person's life more satisfying.

PRIVACY

Privacy is precious to all of us. We like to be able to decide who we tell our secrets to and who knows our business. We like to be able to decide who sees or touches our "private parts." We have private conversations, private correspondence, and private thoughts. And sometimes we just like to be alone, away from intrusions, having a little private time.

If you had a disability that required you to receive support services in a group living situation, you would probably lose a lot of your precious privacy. People would keep notes about your bad behavior, and they might keep a chart of which days you had a BM or when you started your menstrual period. If you needed assistance with bathing or other personal hygiene tasks, a person you didn't choose would be touching your private parts. Someone might monitor your phone calls, or you

Chapter 10 – A Matter of Rights

might have to receive your calls in the living room where the other people you live with are watching TV. If you were learning to dress yourself, the steps of your training program might be posted on the wall of your bedroom, announcing to anyone who comes in that you need help with private tasks. You might not be allowed to close the door to your bedroom unless you request "private time" which everyone in the house knows means time for masturbation. How would you feel if you had to live your life in public in a badly operated group home?

Privacy is a precious commodity in a group living environment. On 127 North Crib, if someone had a dirty diaper, we'd just plunk him down on the floor in front of everyone else and change him. Then we'd call across the room to our co-worker, "Daryl just had a BM. Make sure you mark it on the chart." We never gave it a second thought.

If you work in a place like that, apply Our Standard. How would you like to be treated if you needed assistance with your bath? I'd like to choose the person who gives me that kind of help. I'd like that person to be gentle and respectful. Maybe she could close the shower curtain and just reach through only as much as she needs to. I'd like her to ask me what's alright. "Is it OK if I help you wash your privates?" And if she needs to ask me about personal information, I'd like her to talk in a low voice, so everyone else can't hear.

Privacy also means the opportunity to be away from the constant schedules and programs and demands of group living. I was once consulting at a large group home in an inner city neighborhood. The place was considered so dangerous that female professionals had to request an escort to walk them from their cars to the home. A high security fence surrounded the back yard of the house. At one point during the hectic evening routine of cleaning up after supper, running training programs, and getting baths done, I looked around for Steven, a man I had met earlier in the day. I hadn't seen him for a while, so I asked a staff person if she knew where he was. "Oh, he's probably out back," replied the busy woman, who bustled toward the bathroom, her arms full of clean towels.

I looked out in the back yard, and there was Steven, sitting on the top of the picnic table, smoking his pipe. Though the noises of the urban neighborhood were all around, the view across the security fence was of a pink and orange sunset on that warm summer evening. I asked Steven if it was OK for me to sit with him. He said, "Mmmm." Steven never used words. We sat in the silence for a few minutes and I said, "Nice evening." Steven said, "Mmmm," and grinned around the stem of his pipe. Steven had found his little bit of private space in an otherwise crowded world.

CONFIDENTIALITY

Confidentiality is a little like privacy, but it's not a concern of those of us who live in the real world. Confidentiality is a concern of the world of supports and treatment and service provision.

When you are employed to provide support services to someone, you will be allowed to read her record. Everyone who receives paid services has one. Keeping good records is usually a requirement of receiving funds. That record has the person's diagnosis, her history (usually with more emphasis on the bad things she's done than on her accomplishments), her treatment plan and life goals, the medications she takes, her weight, her frequency of bowel movements and menstrual periods, her dietary needs—in short, a whole bunch of information most of us would consider private.

You get to see that information because she or her legal representative has signed a Release of Information form giving permission for people who work with her to view her confidential (personal and private) information.

This permission puts you under a legal obligation. You are forbidden from re-releasing that information to anyone who is not also granted a release. That means you can't tell your spouse or your neighbor about anything that is in the record. It means you can't make copies of anything in the record. It means that when you are carrying the record you must take steps to see that no unauthorized person sees it. It also means that you are not allowed to talk about any information that is in the record. Even something as seemingly harmless as the names of the people you work with at a particular facility is confidential and cannot be shared. Most states have laws that punish violations of confidentiality with fines or imprisonment or the loss of your job. Confidentiality is a serious matter.

There is a phrase in the self-advocacy movement that says, "Nothing about us without us." It means don't talk *about* us; talk *with* us. It means we want to be there to give (or withhold) our permission when you are exchanging information about us. It means we want you to help us make our own decisions, not just make decisions for us. If you follow that rule, you'll be sure the person you are supporting is the one who decides when and with whom to share personal information.

Privacy and confidentiality are rights that are easily violated and may require creativity on your part to protect. Always make sure you respect people's privacy the way you would want yours respected.

ABUSE AND NEGLECT—IT HURTS EVERYONE

I guess I'm naïve. I'm always surprised when people who are entrusted with the care and support of people with disabilities violate that trust and treat them badly. It does happen, way too often, despite our best attempts at hiring only people with good hearts and high standards.

Sometimes neglect (failure to provide basic support and protection) happens because staff exercise bad judgment or are poorly trained. Abuse can happen when people providing supports get stressed out and take out their bad feelings on the most vulnerable people in their world.

Sometimes, though, we let bad people slip through our hiring practices. Their actions hurt all of us. It is in everyone's interest to keep those people from tearing down everything we work so hard for. It is your moral obligation to recognize abuse and neglect and do everything you can to prevent them. It is your legal responsibility to report any abuse or neglect you witness to the proper authorities. The organization you work for will have procedures about who to report to and how to report. Follow them.

There are no excuses for abuse and neglect. Covering them up hurts everyone.

How do you know if something you see is abuse or neglect? First, you need to know the definition of the various kinds of offenses—

> **Neglect:** any action or absence of action that fails to provide for proper care or treatment in a safe environment—allowing a person to participate in grossly unsafe activities; failure to meet basic needs (food, shelter, clothing, health care); not advocating for a person's rights

Physical Abuse: any act (including encouraging others to act) that results in harm— including spanking, hitting, rough treatment, or unauthorized use of restraints

Psychological/Emotional Abuse: any action or threat that may cause an individual to feel humiliated, embarrassed, scared, or intimidated

Verbal Abuse: any actions (including encouraging others to act) which degrade (put down) or threaten an individual. It may include spoken words, written words, or gestures. It also includes the use of profanity, calling people by inappropriate nicknames, and /or referring to adults with childlike references.

Sexual Abuse: sexual activity of any kind where legal consent is not given. This includes inappropriate touching, exposing of body parts, sexual jokes or suggestions and /or sexual acts. Any sexual contact between an employee of a provider agency and a person receiving services is strictly forbidden, whether consent was present or not.

Don't worry too much about the fine points of a definition. If you truly do this work for the love of it, your behavior should be far from anything even close to abuse or neglect.

Don't worry about definitions, either, when you're deciding what to report. Report what you see if it doesn't seem right or fair and it makes you feel uncomfortable. Report it if it's not the way you would like to be treated. Use Our Standard.

You are not going to have to judge the person accused of abuse. If you report something you think might have been abuse, there will be an investigation of what happened. Everyone is entitled to due process, including someone accused of abuse or neglect. You will tell your story. The accused will tell hers. Witnesses and victims will be interviewed. A group of people with the proper authority will decide whether a person accused of abuse or neglect is guilty and what action should be taken.

When I was the Director of the ECHO Program, two women who worked second shift asked to see me privately in my office. They were both in tears as they described how they had seen one of their co-workers hit a man in the back with her large ring of keys while he was in the shower.

They said, "She does this kind of thing all the time, and we just can't stand it anymore." Their report didn't surprise me. I had had concerns about the accused woman's attitude before, but I had never had enough evidence to get rid of her.

I told the women in my office they were right in coming to me and asked them to each give me a signed written statement of what happened. They got very nervous and said they didn't want to write a statement because they "didn't want to get anyone in trouble." I did my best to keep my supervisory cool and said, "Ladies, you've just reported to me that you witnessed a serious case of physical abuse. If you don't make an official report, I'll have to consider you as guilty as the one who did the hitting." They wrote their statements. I called the perpetrator into my office, asked her for her keys and told her to leave the facility. Some very vulnerable people were safer that night because of that woman's absence.

Don't worry about getting someone in trouble. It is everyone's job to root out abuse and neglect and see that people guilty of it are gotten out of this business. Then we can get on with the more important job of helping people exercise their rights.

GUARDIANSHIP

Most of us, when we become adults, are free to make choices for ourselves. When we agree to do something, it is said we give our "consent." Because we are responsible adults who understand the consequences of our choices, we say our consent is "informed." We'll talk more about the issues of informed consent in the next chapter. For now, it's sufficient to know that a person can give informed consent when they understand the consequences of their decision.

People who cannot understand the consequences of their choices and their behavior may need a guardian to look after their interests. Guardians are appointed by local courts when someone demonstrates that an adult person is not able to give informed consent about some area of his life. There has to be a due process procedure in which the court hears the person and makes a decision on whether he understands the consequences of his decisions. Due process is the safeguard to keep unscrupulous family members or others from taking control over someone's life just for their own convenience or to get control of that person's assets.

If the court rules that the person in question is not able to give informed consent, it is said that he is "adjudicated incompetent." "Incompetent" means "not capable" and "adjudicated" means determined by a judge or court. Once a person is adjudicated incompetent he loses certain of his rights.

Usually the rights that are lost or limited are spelled out in the court document. It is important to realize that adjudication of incompetence and the appointment of a guardian do not necessarily mean the person has no rights to make any decisions in his life anymore. It does not give the guardian the power to run the person's life, only to make decisions in the area where the court has agreed the person needs protection from exploitation.

Unfortunately, in many states, any persons who have a diagnosis of mental retardation (demonstrated by an IQ test score of less than 70) may be automatically declared incompetent as soon as they reach their 18th birthday. Many people have been adjudicated incompetent just because of their disability and with no consideration of whether they in fact are able to make many of the important decisions about their lives.

Often guardians are family members; but family members, unfortunately, do not always have the person's best interests in mind. Sometimes public agency social workers or private agency volunteers (e.g., The Arc) serve as guardians. Some are good at supporting as much choice-making as the person wants; others routinely violate a person's rights and see themselves as in control of the life of the person they are supposed to protect.

When Fred started working at a regular job making minimum wage, he had money in his pocket for the first time in his 24 years. One Friday after being paid, he asked his support staff person to stop at a convenience store so he could buy some stuff. One of the things he bought was a Playboy magazine. When he got back to the group home, he made a point of showing the magazine around in the living room. He was told some people don't like to see that kind of thing, and he reluctantly agreed to keep his magazines in his bedroom. Week after week, the pile of men's magazines under Fred's bed grew. He kept them to himself, and they didn't cause a problem to anyone else in the house.

When it came time for Fred's annual planning meeting, his guardian, a woman who worked for a local agency, attended. When she visited with

Fred in his bedroom, he showed her his stack of magazines. She was upset about them, believing them to be an evil influence on Fred. When we were sitting around the table in the dining room, discussing Fred's goals for the year, the guardian said she wanted the group home staff to take his magazines away from him. I told her we couldn't do that. They were Fred's magazines, and taking them would be a violation of his right to have his own private property. She informed us that as his guardian, she had the power to make all decisions for him. I had a heated argument with her about it and she gave in. But the episode left a bad taste in my mouth about the possibility of guardians violating people's rights rather than protecting them.

GUARDIANSHIP OPTIONS

If a person you are working with is having trouble with a guardian, the first step is for you to look for situations to educate the guardian about rights in general and the person's abilities specifically. Many times guardians don't know about "informed consent," and they think they are responsible for all decisions regarding their ward. If you gently win over their trust, you may help them feel confident about letting their ward make more decisions for herself.

There are alternatives to full guardianship that protect people from exploitation while still upholding their right to make choices in their lives. For example, a guardian *ad litem*, often an attorney, can be selected to protect a person's legal rights. Or a medical guardian could be appointed who would help a person make medical decisions and would sign medical documents giving permission for treatment. Or a trustee can be set up to be guardian over the person's estate, making sure no one takes her property. Advocacy organizations such as The Arc have a lot of good information on alternatives to guardianship. You can contact them through the references in the Resources section of this book.

If the guardian is abusive or negligent in any way, you can help the ward petition for a reassignment of guardianship. This will get him a new guardian who might be more supportive of his rights.

Finally, if you believe the person you are working with has been wrongly adjudicated incompetent or has developed enough skills to be able to have her decision making rights restored, you can help her petition for restoration of competence.

Many self-advocates are now going through the legal process of having their competency restored. It is very rewarding to see a person who used to live in an institution but who now has a job and his own apartment, stand before the judge and ask to be considered a full citizen again.

Larry was a man who couldn't stay still. When I first met him at a self-advocacy conference he was a noticeable presence in almost every session. He strode quickly into a room, looked around to see who was there and what was happening, then moved on, as if on some righteous quest. There was one session, though, where he stayed in place. That was because his place was behind the speaker's table. Larry had been chosen to speak on the issue of restoration of competence.

When the lawyers were finished with their comments, Larry grabbed the microphone and nervously stood to address the audience. He told of the many years when "to tell you the truth, I wasn't doing too good." He admitted he'd had his share of run-ins with authority. He described his many years of institutionalization as a time when "they were trying to make me do right." But the highlight of his remarks was when he described how, with the help of the aforementioned lawyers, he had gone to the court to tell the judge that he had "straightened myself out." He told the judge that he had a good job that he'd stayed at for over a year. He had his own apartment and hadn't been in trouble. In short, he had worked hard to become a responsible adult.

It was a great day in Larry's life when the judge signed the papers that said, "I'm my own man." What does Larry think about petitioning the court to have your rights restored? "I'd recommend it," he says, with a wide grin.

Larry was acting like a responsible adult and so had the rights and privileges of one. But what does that mean, to be a responsible adult? In the next chapter we'll take a closer look at some of the issues.

Chapter 11

SEX, SMOKES AND THE RESPONSIBLE ADULT

EXERCISING RIGHTS

It's not enough to just protect people's rights. That's still the "do for" mentality. When you make sure a person is free from abuse and neglect and exploitation, you're doing a good job taking care of that person. But protection doesn't teach a person how to use the rights you are protecting for him. You have to go beyond protection into advocacy, the active support of a person exercising his rights.

When a person learns to exercise his rights in a way that does not hurt or limit the rights of others, he is finally learning to be a responsible adult. He will then be accepted in the real world with the rest of us responsible adults.

The first step in helping a person exercise her rights is to make sure she knows what her rights are. Many people with disabilities will understand their rights if they are simply told about them. You can use the material in Chapter 10 as a basis for explaining a person's rights to him. Maybe your organization publishes a Rights Handbook for the people you support. You can go through this kind of material with a person who is learning about her rights, explaining unfamiliar words and answering questions.

Remember, though, that many people learn best by participating. They might not understand a word of the Rights Handbook, but they could learn a lot by attending a self-advocacy group meeting. Experienced self-advocates are always willing to bring someone new into the exciting world of speaking up for your rights. You could spend a day watching court procedures and talking about due process. You might attend a county commissioner's meeting when they're discussing funding for mental health services.

The right to choose little things in our lives is a very basic right that people who have lived in institutional environments may not know how to exercise. The simplest way for a person to learn that she has basic rights like deciding what to eat and when to go to bed is to ask her what she would like. That's really helping her exercise the right, not just telling her that she has that right. You teach a lot about rights by respecting them.

Sometimes people have no interest in exercising particular rights. Lots of people don't vote, for instance. How can you know which rights the person you're working with wants to exercise? If you've been paying attention, your answer should come quickly—"Ask him." And what if he doesn't talk? He'll tell you with his behavior. Give him opportunities to exercise rights and see if he's interested.

RESPONSIBILITIES

Many lifetimes ago, when I was a Religious Education Director, I taught a Sunday School class about "Rights and Responsibilities." The class was for fifth graders and was about how if you want to have rights, you've got to accept responsibilities. I liked the way those two were balanced in the curriculum—rights and responsibilities. You can't have one without the other.

You probably already know that rights and responsibilities go together. That's because you're an adult who has been living a real life in the real world. You've learned that rights are the things you are permitted to do and that responsibilities are the limits you have to accept in order to keep your rights from violating the rights of others. Responsibilities are the price of living in a social world. You've also learned that if you act in an irresponsible manner, you may lose your rights. Like I said before, you can't have one without the other.

People who have lived in institutional environments where their rights have been routinely violated may not have learned this balance of rights and responsibilities. The institution takes on the responsibility of caring for the person. The staff set behavioral boundaries for people and make sure no one makes mistakes or gets into trouble. The price for someone else taking responsibility for your life is the loss of your rights. As I said earlier, if I'm going to be responsible for you, I'm probably not going to let you exercise your right to run your own life.

INFORMED CONSENT

Why do care-taking institutions take on the responsibility for the lives of people with disabilities? Because they believe those people cannot be responsible for their own lives. They believe people with disabilities will do stupid things, make mistakes, hurt themselves, or fail to reach their goals—just like we all do. The difference is that our failures are tolerated because we're seen as being responsible for ourselves. If someone else takes responsibility for your life (because of a disability) you may lose your right to be a sloppy, sometimes failing human being like everybody else.

There are, of course, some people who truly are not held responsible, legally or morally, for their actions. That is because these people are so disabled in their decision making functions that they don't understand the consequences of their choices. It then becomes someone else's responsibility to keep them safe and to make decisions for them in a way that is believed to be in their best interest. We discussed that in the "Guardianship" section of Chapter 10.

How do you tell the difference between the person who needs to be supported to become a responsible adult in the real world and the one who needs a supportive guardian to make sure her best interests are served? The answer lies in the concept of "informed consent."

"Informed consent" means the person has and understands the information needed to say "yes" (consent) to a certain course of action. It doesn't mean that he made the same decision you would make or the same decision his case manager would make. It doesn't mean he will always choose the "right" way to go and never make a mistake. All informed consent means is that the person understands the possible consequences of his decisions and actions.

It's really quite simple—someone who doesn't understand what might happen cannot know how to avoid danger and has to be protected.

Someone who does understand the consequences is free to choose what she wants to do...even if some people think her choices are stupid or dangerous.

Let's take sex, for example (You did come to this chapter for the sex, didn't you?). What if you are working with a 28-year-old woman who doesn't speak, who gets lost if she gets out of sight of her home, and who needs assistance in even the most basic personal tasks? You have a little sex education class with her, using anatomically correct dolls and all the necessary charts and diagrams. When you ask her to point at any body part, she always points at the male doll's penis. You have informed her about pregnancy and sexually transmitted diseases, but you found out from the nurse that this woman can't even tell staff if she feels sick. You tried to get her to sit in on a group discussion of dating practices, but she sneaked into the kitchen and ate a bag of cookies. Do you think this woman can give informed consent to intercourse with another adult man who is interested? She has been informed. You told her everything she needs to know. If she doesn't resist, doesn't that mean she consents? Of course not. It is clear this woman does not understand the consequences of her decisions and therefore cannot give informed consent.

On the other hand, let's look at Tony. Tony is also an adult who has a developmental disability, but he speaks plenty. He considers himself the Don Juan of the sheltered workshop where he works. He dresses flamboyantly and claims to have had sex with hundreds of women. He was in the discussion group about dating, and he wasn't interested in the cookies. He was interested in Betty, the woman who was running the group. He has had several instructional classes in sex education. He can demonstrate the correct use of a condom, knows where babies come from, and knows more about sexually transmitted diseases than many of his home staff. He also realizes a lot of people think badly of someone who has sex with a lot of different partners. But he doesn't care about that. He's ready to "do it" with anyone who's willing. Can he give informed consent? I think so. He understands the consequences of his behavior. We may think his behavior is risky and stupid. We may even think it is immoral. We're entitled to our opinions. But we're not entitled to make decisions for someone who is capable of making them for himself.

Everyone has the right to do stupid things, as long as they understand the consequences. People who smoke cigarettes, for example, surely know that smoking is bad for them. But they do it anyway. They are adults who give informed consent.

If you went to your doctor's office for a check-up, and the doctor said you're 50 pounds overweight and are running a high risk of a heart attack, have you been informed? Yes; and you fully understand the information you were given. You're an adult who is capable of informed consent. You'd sure be shocked if later that evening the doctor showed up at your house and took away your ice cream! You might show the doctor some challenging behavior.

It is not your job to take away people's opportunity to have sex, smoke cigarettes, be overweight, or any number of other risky things, as long as you can show that they understand the consequences of their behavior. It is your job, instead, to try to motivate them to engage in behaviors that are more likely to bring them what they want and less likely to cause trouble. It's an issue of teaching, not of control.

Norman had been told, by his mother and his doctor, that he should quit smoking. His years as a street alcoholic and his repeated admissions to the state psychiatric hospital meant that, at the age of 65, Norman was in chronic poor health. The smoking only made it worse.

Norman's mother, who was in her late eighties, was his guardian. Many of my colleagues on Norman's support team felt that if the doctor and the guardian ordered Norman to quit smoking it was our job to enforce the doctor's orders. I disagreed. I had talked with Norman about it. He knew that smoking was bad for him; but he said it was "the only G—D— thing I've got left in my life, and I'm gonna die soon, anyway." I had heard some of my smoking co-workers say almost the same thing. I suggested to the team that we might take a different approach.

I talked with Norman, in private, just before we were going to have the "house meeting" on what to do about his smoking. I said, "Norman, you know your doctor and your mother are worried that your smoking is going to make you sick or kill you."

"Yeah, I know," he replied, "but I ain't gonna quit."

"I know that," I said. "But the cigarettes are getting pretty expensive, too. Do you think you might be able to cut down some? I think that would make your mama happy, and you'd save a little money that you could spend on coffee when we go to Hardees. You could still smoke, but not as many."

Norman thought about that a bit and said, "I guess I might cut down a little."

I asked him, "How many cigarettes do you think you would need every day?" He was currently smoking about a pack a day.

He thought about that a long time. He was seriously trying to figure how many he'd need. When you talk this way with a person who has difficulty thinking, you have to be patient and let him come up with his own answer. He said, "I think maybe eight."

That was less than I'd thought. But always "take what you can get closest to what you want." I jumped at it. "Eight would be great, Norman."

He grinned and said "'Eight would be great.' You made a poem."

"Yeah, I guess I did." I wanted to be sure he hadn't gotten distracted. "But let me make sure I understand what you're agreeing to—eight cigarettes a day."

"Yeah," he replied. "Eight would be great." I had already worked with Norman on how important it is to "honor your word," so he held out his hand, and we shook on it.

I still wasn't satisfied he had really given informed consent. I felt I needed to go into more detail with him. I asked him, "Is there something we could do to help you stick with only eight cigarettes a day? Can you carry a whole pack of cigarettes in your pocket and only smoke eight in a day? Or would you maybe like us to give you eight cigarettes each day and keep the rest of them for you?"

I was hitting him with a little too many choices, so I let him have time to think. He said, "Well, if I carry 'em all, I'll just smoke 'em all." I thought that was pretty good insight for a person who was supposed to not be able to make any decisions for himself.

I pressed on. "If we keep your cigarettes for you, would it be better if we gave them to you at certain times of the day? Or half in the morning and half in the evening?"

More thinking from Norman. "Well, I don't want no smoke schedule where they tell me," (he goes into a sing-song controlling whine he's heard from staff) 'No, Norman, you can't have a cigarette until 4:00.'" Apparently Norman was experienced with this sort of thing. "I want to carry 'em myself and smoke 'em when I want to."

Take what you can get, remember? "OK," I replied, "how about if we give you four in the morning and four in the afternoon. That way you won't smoke them all at once and have to go all day without." He thought that was a great idea. In fact, he understood the idea of our helping him discipline himself so well that he added a little wrinkle of his own. "You know," he said, "I always like to have one right before I go to bed. So how about if you hold one back, so I'll always have one at bedtime." I said that was perfect and told him how much I appreciated his working with me on this.

We then went to the house meeting and I had Norman tell the staff what he had agreed to and what he wanted them to do to help him meet the terms of his agreement.

Norman left our meeting feeling empowered. He was doing something good for his health and pleasing his doctor and his mother. He was not, however, giving over control of his life to some do-good professionals. He was acting like a responsible adult. He kept the right to change his mind and go back to his old smoking rate. And he could have decided not to cut down in the first place. Responsible adults get to do stupid things.

LEARNING TO BE A RESPONSIBLE ADULT

When people get out of an institutional life and start living in the community with the rest of us, they are often told that they now have rights. They are seldom told that they also have responsibilities.

The result is people who are puffed up about doing whatever they want to do, whenever they feel like it. "I have my rights." Is it surprising that some citizens will experience these new neighbors as irresponsible and dangerous? Is it surprising that these newborn rights advocates don't want to keep a job if it requires commitment, are inconsiderate of their neighbors, and can act abusively in relationships? They've never been taught that rights and responsibilities are part of the same package. They've never been taught how to be what we call a "responsible adult."

I have often had to teach people who spent many years in institutional environments what it means to be a responsible adult. I teach five rules:

Honor your word
The institutional mindset believes, "What they don't know won't hurt them." The staff have information; the residents don't. This is often based on the common attitude toward people with mental retardation that "They don't understand it, anyway." Lies of convenience are justified as keeping good order.

People who've lived in such settings don't know that in the real world nobody much likes a liar. They don't know that you have to earn people's trust by doing what you say you're going to do. They have to learn to honor their word.

Let's say I want Jorge to make a commitment about working. I say, "Jorge, if I help you get this job that you want, you've got to promise to work as hard as you can and do everything the boss tells you to do. Can you agree to that?" Jorge says he sure can. I get him to repeat the agreement so I know he understood it. I then say, looking him in the eye, "OK, let's shake on it." We shake hands and the deal is sealed.

A week later, when Jorge wants to lay down on the job because the boss is too bossy, I remind him of his agreement to follow the boss' instructions. "A responsible adult," I say, "honors his word." He recalls our handshake and backs off from his resistance, saying proudly, "That's right. I'm a man of my word." Jorge has learned one piece of his responsibility as a citizen of the real world.

Follow the rules
We all have to follow rules. We stop when the light is red and go when it's green. We don't urinate in public. When we start a new job, we receive an employee handbook that tells all the rules for attendance, how to dress, and how to act on the job. Most of these rules are fair and are applied to everyone. We follow these rules because we know they help everyone get along.

A person who has lived in an institutional world has been subjected to rules that he had no say in and that are applied only to people like him, people who are not equal to the staff who make the rules. When he gets out of the institution and learns he has rights, he thinks that means he now doesn't have to follow any rules.

The best way to show this person the necessity of following rules is to show the ways *you* have to follow rules. Look for opportunities to show what would happen in our real world if everyone acted irresponsibly and, instead of following rules, just did whatever they felt like doing. Littering might be a good example. Spend a day out cleaning up roadside trash as part of an Adopt-a-Highway program and the person you're working with will soon be fuming about why these people can't follow the rules.

Follow procedures

Part of growing up into a responsible adult is learning the ways to get things done. There are procedures for everything.

Submit a form, call a meeting, take two steps back and hold your mouth right. We have learned to follow the procedures that get us what we want. That's why people do what they do, remember? To get what they want.

If a person has learned that the way to get out of doing a task he doesn't want to do is to raise a ruckus, that's what he'll do at work when the job moves too fast for him. You have to help him see that "there's a better way of doing this." Then show him how to make a suggestion or address a grievance...following procedures.

I have had good results helping people in group living situations learn that there is a team of people who are there to support their success. If they want something changed in their life, they need to ask for a meeting of the team and work with them to bring about the change. A couple of times of this being successful is all it takes.

I remember when Jerry and Mickey decided to test this team thing. They called a team meeting, saying they wanted to discuss something with us. We assembled around the dining room table at their home. They told us, barely suppressing their smirks, they had decided what they really wanted from the team was girlfriends and alcohol. The team told Jerry and Mickey that it was not the team's job to provide those things for them. We might, though, be able to help them achieve their goals themselves. For instance, we could provide them with the opportunity to have increasing amounts of unsupervised time, during which they could do whatever they wanted. The price of the free time would be showing that they could use it responsibly, that is, without getting into trouble. Jerry and Mickey agreed to our proposal and suggested some details of the plan.

We started out with 15 minutes unsupervised time at a local town street fair. They were both back at the appointed place at the appointed time, so the time was increased. Gradually, they both worked up to being able to have overnight unsupervised time, at which time they were ready to live on their own...and do as they pleased.

Following the procedure for getting things done had worked for them, and they continued to go through the channels that worked, as they found their way to independence.

Treat others fairly and with respect

Did you ever notice how people sometimes get the Golden Rule backwards? You're supposed to treat other people the way you would like them to treat you. But some people think the rule means you should treat other people the way they have treated you in the past. It's a formula for revenge. It justifies bad behavior because the other guy did it first.

People who have been treated disrespectfully and unfairly have a lot of anger stored up. They come into the community ready to do unto others the way they've been done unto.

We have to help them turn that around. We have to help them understand that in our world you earn respect by being respectful.

The best way to teach someone fairness and respect is by acting that way toward them and by insisting they return the favor. Sometimes what I call "straight talk" is the most respectful thing you can do. When the person you are supporting calls you names or puts you down, you look the person in the eye and say, "I don't talk to you like that, and I expect you not to talk to me that way either." You are demonstrating that fairness and respect are a two way street—if you want them, you have to give them.

Accept natural consequences

A "natural consequence" is what naturally follows a particular behavior in the real world. We all learn appropriate behavior by experiencing the natural consequences of our actions. Some kinds of actions get us what we want, and some kinds of actions bring us pain and sorrow. Natural consequences are the way the real world works.

Sometimes people who have lived in institutional settings have been protected from natural consequences. When Frank came up to a female staff person at the state hospital, put his arms around her and said, "Hey, baby, how about it?" she probably just laughed and said, "Frank, I'm not your girlfriend today." When he does the same thing to the attractive girl in line at McDonald's, her boyfriend, who is just returning from the restroom, is likely to threaten to punch Frank's lights out. Of course, I don't want Frank to get hurt, but I wouldn't mind his being scared a little. I'm not going to rescue him from a powerful lesson in social behavior.

These are just some of the lessons in learning to become a responsible adult. It's not easy. Sometimes those of us who work hard and follow the rules look like the foolish ones. We're exhausted and burned out, while the people we support are happy with a roof over their heads and a fresh pack of cigarettes every day. They are being taken care of, but they may not realize the extent to which their freedom is taken away. We choose to try to be responsible adults because we know that's the way we can make our own decisions and live our own lives.

I'll never forget the time Willie said to me, in anger and frustration, "James, sometimes I don't care about being a responsible adult!" I had to sympathize. Sometimes I don't care about being a responsible adult, either. But I continue to try to be one because I know the rewards it brings. I know how good it feels to be a respected member of a community. I want the Willies of this world to know that good feeling, too.

THE SEX PART

I know, you've been waiting for this part. And I've made you read through all this stuff about responsibility and rights and informed consent.

You've seen how people with disabilities have the same rights as everyone else. You've seen how we dealt with Norman's smoking as an issue of supporting responsibility and informed consent. Now let's apply what you've learned to the issue of the sexual expression of people with disabilities.

Sexuality is important because it is an area where the rights of people with disabilities who live in segregated environments are routinely violated. That's right, I said "routinely," as in every day, all the time, without even giving it a second thought.

Adults with disabilities are often placed in group homes where it is "against the rules" to have your boyfriend or girlfriend visit you privately in your room.

Adults with disabilities are sometimes appointed guardians who decide, "I don't want her to have sex." Then they make the support provider agency responsible to make sure she doesn't.

All kinds of excuses are used to keep people with disabilities from having sex. You will hear that it is against the law in your state or province for unmarried people to have sex. At the same time, many of your co-workers are involved in non-marital or extra-marital affairs, and the police are not breaking down their bedroom doors.

You will hear that the group home where you work is "responsible for" the people who live there. You cannot, therefore, allow people to have sexual relationships, because they might lead to disease or unwanted pregnancy. Your organization would then be liable and get sued. Do you recall what I said earlier about how taking responsibility for someone takes away their rights? This is a perfect example.

SOURCES OF DISCOMFORT

"Children in adult bodies"
Sexuality in people with disabilities is an issue that causes a great deal of discomfort in a lot of people. Sometimes this discomfort is the result of people thinking someone who has mental retardation is really "a child in an adult body." We wouldn't let two five-year-olds have private sex in their bedroom. So why should we allow such activity to a person we think of as having "the mind of a five-year-old?"

One way to deal with the perception that people with disabilities are children is to come back to the issue of informed consent. If a person is over the age of 18 and understands the consequences of his decision, he should be supported in following through on that decision. If he cannot understand the consequences of his decision, he should be protected from harm. We are indeed responsible for helping people avoid exploitation and abuse. If they don't understand what is happening to them, we need to protect them.

We are also responsible for seeing that people understand the consequences of their decisions. We can help them get the information and experience they need.

But we are not responsible for keeping people from experiencing the full richness of life, including life as a sexual being.

Deviant and dangerous
Another reason people shy away from supporting people with disabilities to be fully expressive sexually is that some people equate mental retardation with sexual deviance. They think people who have developmental disabilities also have weird sexual tastes or are sexual predators. Where do they get these ideas? Well, their knowledge is often limited to what they see on TV or hear about through the grapevine. The "retarded man" who was caught masturbating naked in the bushes behind someone's house gets full, excited coverage on the six o'clock news. The couple with disabilities who have a long term loving partnership are unnoticed.

If we gave people with disabilities the same opportunity to explore and express their sexuality that everyone else has, I suspect they would show "deviant" sexual behavior at about the same rate as our other friends and neighbors. There would be people with disabilities who prefer relationships with the same sex. There would be people with disabilities who prefer solitary masturbation or pornography or cross-dressing. There would be people with disabilities who are peeping toms or sexual predators.

The problem is that people who have lived in institutions don't have the same opportunity to explore and express their sexuality. Institutional restrictions bend people out of shape. By not allowing and supporting full sexual expression in the context of loving relationships, the institution warps people's sexuality. Then we use the warped-ness to justify further restrictions. You can't win for losing.

"That's disgusting"
I was once training a group of potential foster parents. These couples were going to have to work with some pretty difficult teenagers and

young adults, so I always told horror stories in training. I wanted to scare away the squeamish ones.

One evening I told of a man who always masturbated when he was upset or anxious, no matter where he was or who else was present. I was trying to help the group identify their own hang-ups and learn creative ways of dealing with challenging behavior. At one of the breaks, a woman came up to me and said in a whisper, "I don't think I'm going to be able to do this." I asked her why not. She replied, "Well, you know that thing you were talking about that that man did?"

"You mean 'masturbate'?" I asked, knowing full well what she was talking about.

She shuddered and turned red. Gulping for air, she said, "Yes...well, I can't even think about it. It's so disgusting."

I was glad she recognized her reaction. I told her she was probably right in feeling she wouldn't be able to be a supportive foster parent. If you think something a person does is disgusting, you probably won't be able to support them to be fully who they are.

Some people think the very notion of a person with a disability having sex is disgusting. The very idea of needing support with activities that are usually so personal and private turns many people off. How would you feel, for instance, if a person you supported wanted to go to a prostitute who specialized in working with people with disabilities? Could you help a person buy an inflatable sex doll or a vibrator? Do you think people who can learn no other way should be taught masturbation techniques through physical assistance? These are some of the serious issues that are raised when we commit to fully supporting people. Some of the pioneers in our field, people like Winifred Kempton and David Hingsburger, have been attacked and insulted for their courageous support of full sexuality for people with disabilities. It takes courage to break new ground and open new opportunities. You'll never be able to do it if your personal objections get in the way.

HOW DO WE SUPPORT SEXUAL EXPRESSION?

I wrote the sexuality policy we used at Access, Inc. It said we supported any sexual behavior that:
- Is done alone or with a legally consenting, age-appropriate partner
- Occurs at an appropriate time and in an appropriate place
- Is within the limits permitted by law and societal norms

I was fudging a little when I used the word "appropriate." This is a word that has been used as a club to beat up on any behavior the controlling majority doesn't like or feel comfortable with. They say, "Stop doing that. It's inappropriate." In this case, though, we do have social norms for how much age difference is appropriate in a sexual relationship. The law cuts a lot more slack to the 15-year-old boy who has sex with a 14-year-old girl than it does to a 30-year-old man with the same girl. And "appropriate time and place" are meant to address issues of privacy and respect for others that arise in group living situations. You can't have sex on the couch if your roommate is trying to watch TV. Just be careful if you use "appropriate" to describe sexual behavior that you're not using a "special" standard applied only to people who have disabilities.

The organization you work for probably has a written policy about sexual matters. I hope it supports people's rights.

If we want to change the current situation, we have to do three things:

- Provide information about sex and relationships (sex education)
- Support the development of intimate relationships for people who have been denied them
- Educate the community at large that people with disabilities have the same rights of sexual expression as everyone else

SEX EDUCATION

The first task is "sex education." This should more appropriately be called "relationship education" or "being-an-adult-human-being education." Such education needs to:

- give people the information they need,

- answer their questions and clear up misunderstandings,
- and be accepting of personal differences.

GIVE PEOPLE THE INFORMATION THEY NEED

I have been involved with sex education courses (for "normal" teenagers, as well as for people with disabilities) that mostly conveyed clinical information and terminology. There's nothing wrong with those things. I guess I'm glad I know where the Fallopian tubes are, though I've never seen one. And I've certainly never had a relationship with one.

The problem with this kind of sex education for people with disabilities is the same problem I have with other training programs that don't really address a person's need to know. People who have mental retardation have trouble learning things. So we don't need to clutter their minds with the Latin names of the 16 parts of the female genitalia. Sex education classes should be structured to respond to the real needs and questions of the people in the class. That means the environment must be comfortable, accepting, and flexible. Sometimes that isn't a "class" at all. It's just the kind of stuff that comes up when you develop relationships that are trustworthy and caring.

Many people with disabilities (a majority, according to some studies) have been sexually abused. They have been hurt in the physical and emotional areas you want to teach about in a sex education class. You have to be sensitive to this. Go slow. And when painful questions come up, recognize how privileged you are to be asked about something that may be deeply personal and painful to the person asking. A comfortable, accepting environment is the only place people will talk about what they really need to know or what's really bothering them.

The best sex education usually happens as a "teachable moment." Teachable moments are not on the schedule. They just arise when a person has a question or wants to learn something new. You need to be responsive to teachable moments about sex and relationships. Just be careful you don't answer more than is asked. Too much information can just add to the confusion.

You may have heard the story about the little girl who asked her mother, "Where did I come from?" Her mother, seeing this as the teachable moment she had been expecting, launched into a lecture about eggs, sperm and conception. The little girl looked puzzled, so Mom asked her, "Did that answer your question?" The girl responded, "Well, I don't know. My best friend said she came from Ohio."

ANSWER THEIR QUESTIONS AND CLEAR UP MISUNDERSTANDINGS

Many people with disabilities have been taught myths and gross misinformation in order to keep them from "doing it." One man was taught you got sick "if you let the white stuff come out." So he masturbated constantly, but never to completion. Staff treated it as a problem and made him wear coveralls that were pinned in the back so he couldn't get into them. One woman was taught that her genital area was "God's place." She protected it as sacred...until she was molested by a clergyman.

Misinformation is never protective. Knowledge is power. If people do not understand their sexuality, they will not be able to give (or withhold) informed consent. Or they will act in ways that the community considers weird and will be segregated again. We must be willing to talk openly about sexual desires, regardless of the form they take. The bright light of information is the best way to protect people from exploitation. It is also the best way to support them to live a real (sexual) life in the real world.

ACCEPTING OF PERSONAL DIFFERENCES

When it comes to issues of sexuality and intimate relationships, we all bring extra baggage with us. We have hang-ups, fears, and pockets of ignorance, moral judgments, and private desires. We can't deny those things. They are part of who we are. The point is not to add the weight of our baggage to the burdens already carried by people with disabilities.

Dave Hingsburger tells a wonderful story about a man with a disability who shouted at him (after what Dave thought was a brilliant sex education session), "You're trying to teach us to do it the way you do it...and that's not the way we do it!" Of course, everyone "does it" differently. That's because we're individuals. It's why we're compatible partners with some people and not with others. The man was telling Dave to listen, to pay attention to the people he supports rather than being the expert. If you want to truly be responsive to people's real needs, you have to keep your Beginner's Mind.

Personal differences are why there is even sex and love at all. If we were all clones of each other, if we all liked the same things and were good at the same things, had the same gifts and gaps, what would be the point of getting together? The problem is that some differences are celebrated, while others are put down and held in contempt. Physical disabilities, in particular, are often seen as making a person less attractive and desirable.

You should know, though, that there are differences that "make a difference." Some disabilities affect how a person functions sexually. If a person you support has physical disabilities that make some kinds of sexual activity difficult, you should help him or her be in touch with people who know how to overcome the particular obstacles they're facing. You also may need to help someone get more information on genetic counseling, so they can make an informed decision about whether to have children. There are many sources in Appendix II: Resources.

Actually, the best "sex education" is not a class and it's not just about sex. It's a community of supportive and caring people who are knowledgeable about sexual and relationship issues. It's people who are dedicated to supporting social growth and a full range of sexual expression for everyone. It's people like you.

SUPPORTING INTIMATE RELATIONSHIPS

Sex isn't just about what people do with their genitals. It's about who we are as men and women. It's about falling in (and out of) love. It's about feeling attractive and valued and worthy. It's about families and children and being part of something bigger than ourselves. Our sexuality, though sometimes the cause of painful and puzzling problems, is also the source of some of our greatest joy and satisfaction.

How would you feel if you were cut off from the opportunity to express yourself fully as a man or a woman? What if people never considered that you might be seen as attractive and desirable? Can you imagine how devastating it would be to know that many people would think it was a tragedy if someone in their family fell in love with you? How empowered could you be if you realized you were seen as the bottom rung of the ladder of attractiveness, an ugly freak, a sexless child?

What if your only intimate time was masturbating alone in a room at a time scheduled for that purpose?

What about having babies? Are you ready to help the people you support make decisions about having and raising children? You'll need to help them learn about the chances of their disability being passed to their children. If their condition is likely to be inherited, you'll have to talk about whether it's really such a bad thing. If I have Down syndrome and I think I'm a pretty good and valuable person, why would I not want to have a son or daughter who's like me? And when you talk about child-raising, you'll have to be honest about what skills are necessary to be a good parent. Do you really have to be able to read and do math, or is it more important that you know how to protect and nurture someone? If my language isn't very good, should I not have a child because I won't be able to teach him to speak? Can't I get some help with that?

We humans thrive on intimate relationships. We love to fall in love. We generally choose to go through life with a partner, even a series of partners, rather than going it alone. Even if we choose to live alone, we have a network of friends and family who care about us, who check up on us when we're sick and want us to call them as soon as we find out if we got the new job. People with disabilities are no different.

Many people think people with disabilities will only be exploited and abused in intimate relationships, not that they would have something to add. They do have something to add. You know that, because you understand everyone is gifted. You know it because you've taken the time to see.

The issues of intimate relationships for people with disabilities can be complicated and tricky. That's one of the reasons many people tend to avoid the whole matter. But I don't think we can let ourselves off the hook. Love and sex and marriage and family are so important to us as human beings that to deny them to people because of a disability is the worst sort of injustice.

EDUCATING THE COMMUNITY AT LARGE

One organization that provides services for people with disabilities decided to get out of the group home business and let people live where and with whom they wanted. This bold decision brought many challenges. For instance, when one woman was asked if she wanted to live alone or with a roommate, she replied that she wanted to live with "George." When asked who George was, she answered, "He's my boyfriend. He works at the workshop." Well, George wasn't even a "client" of the agency. What were they going to do? The answer was that they had to really support what people wanted in their lives. They had to think outside the box. The result was that within three years of their turning everyone loose, half the people they supported were married. Does that surprise you? Isn't marriage one of the ways many of us choose to make our lives less burdensome and more richly satisfying? In this particular instance, the agency even made public service TV ads in which couples who had disabilities gave sound marriage advice to the community. It's amazing what can happen when you trust people and treat them like fully human beings.

We've already seen that the reason many people in our communities have negative images of people with disabilities is that they haven't really seen or known them. You have the opportunity to be an ambassador of goodwill. You can show what the people you support can do. And you can help them learn to speak out for themselves, to be self-advocates.

Chapter 12

DISABILITIES THROUGH THE LIFECYCLE

One thing we all have in common as human beings is that we are born, we grow up, and, if we're lucky, we grow old. We go through times when we feel on top of the world, successful and happy and ready for the future. And there are times when it seems like we don't know anything, when everything seems difficult and dangerous.

We can identify with the person who has disabilities if we think of how we felt during the "terrible twos" or "terrible teens" or "terrible teeterings" (the crisis of growing older), all times when who we are changes. In these times of change, our reach often exceeds our grasp. We get scared and fall back into ourselves. We may not understand what's going on. Much of what we try ends up in failure. People get mad at us. This must be a lot of what it is like to have a mental disability.

If you are supporting a person with disabilities there are some specific things to look for at different times in the lifecycle. Being aware of some of the issues of early childhood, school years, and aging will help you offer the support a person needs and may not be able to ask for.

IN OUR GENES

Back in Chapter 5 we talked about the fact that "developmental" disabilities are the result of something that happens to a person some time "from conception until adulthood." Then we dealt with some of the causes of developmental disabilities. We divided the causes into three timeframes—before birth, during birth, and after birth.

Many advances have been made in understanding what cause disabilities to occur before a person is even born. One area of increased understanding is in genetics. Genetics is the study of how information about who we are going to be is passed down from our parents and how that information is used to assemble all the billions of complicated connections that go into making a human being.

Each of us is different from others (with the exception of identical twins). We got part of the information that formed us from our mothers and part from our fathers. The information that tells cells how to develop is carried in our DNA. The DNA is made up of two sets of chromosomes. We get 23 chromosomes from our mothers and another 23 from our fathers. The chromosomes are made of smaller units called genes. Altogether we each have around 100,000 genes that carry the information for the development of each of our 100 trillion cells. It's amazing that all of these complicated instructions can assemble a fully functioning human being!

Occasionally, though, something goes wrong in the system. For some reason that we don't understand yet, a piece of the instructions for making the developing child can be damaged or missing. The damaged bit of instruction (called a "mutation") causes cells to develop in ways that are very different from the usual way. Sometimes mutations cause some wonderful new ability. After all, it was through millions of years of these "accidents" that human beings developed our big brains and capable hands and sensitive emotions. Some mutations, though, can cause chronic health problems and the kinds of problems with thinking, communication, and learning that are associated with mental retardation.

One of the most common conditions caused by genetic mutation is Down syndrome. As I said above, most people have 23 pairs of chromosomes (for a total of 46), a complete set from each parent. People with Down syndrome have an extra 21st chromosome (which is why the condition is sometimes called "Trisomy 21"). This extra chromosome causes a number of changes in the developing fetus, some of which can be seen at birth. Babies with Down syndrome have certain facial characteristics in common. They also tend to have low muscle tone and excessively flexible joints. And most children with Down syndrome have some degree of developmental delay. They develop new skills more slowly than normal, and they may test in the mild to moderate range of mental retardation. All of these differences from the norm are caused by the extra chromosome.

Some of the other conditions caused by genetic changes (listed from most common to least common) are:

> **Fragile X syndrome**—A defect of the X chromosome which causes mild mental retardation. Occurs more frequently and severely among males than females. The leading known inherited (passed down from the parents) cause of mental retardation in the United States. Symptoms: Language delays, behavioral problems, autism or autistic-like behavior (including poor eye contact and hand-flapping), and enlarged external genitalia.
>
> **Duchenne Muscular Dystrophy**—A hereditary degenerative disease of skeletal (voluntary) muscles, is the most common form of childhood muscular dystrophy. It is usually first identified in children age three to six years. Starting with muscle weakness and wasting in the pelvic area, the disease gradually involves most major muscle groups of the body.
>
> **Trisomy 13 syndrome**—Similar to Down syndrome, this condition is caused by an extra chromosome, this time occurring at chromosome 13. Many infants with Trisomy 13 syndrome fail to grow and gain weight at the expected rate (failure to thrive) and have severe feeding difficulties, reduced muscle tone (hypotonia), and episodes in which breathing stops temporarily (apnea). Life-threatening complications may develop during infancy or early childhood.
>
> **Tuberous Sclerosis**—Usually apparent shortly after birth. Signs of the disorder include: seizures, mental retardation, distinctive skin abnormalities (lesions), and non-cancerous, tumor-like nodules of the brain, certain regions of the eyes, the heart, the kidneys, the lungs, or other tissues or organs.
>
> **Phenylketonuria** (PKU)—Can be inherited from parents. The genetic misinformation causes the newborn child to be unable to process phenylalanine (a protein that is found in all protein foods such as meat, eggs, fish, milk and cheese). If untreated, toxins build up in the newborn's body and can cause severe mental retardation, seizures and other symptoms. The incidence of PKU in developed nations is now greatly reduced because a blood test is given each infant at birth. If the newborn tests positive for PKU, he/she is put on a special diet that reduces or eliminates the damage.
>
> *Adapted from information provided by the National Organization for Rare Disorders (www.rarediseases.org)*

The rapidly growing information in the field of genetics seems to, as the fund raisers say, "offer hope to millions." Every day on TV and in magazines we see new stories of "discovering the gene for" this condition or that. Hope is held out that one day we will recognize the cause of every "birth defect" so that all babies are born "perfect." You know by now that my putting so many words in quotes means I am disturbed by something underlying the way apparently simple terms are being used.

Everyone wants every baby to be born healthy. And we would all like there to be some prevention or cure of some terrible conditions that bring enormous suffering and pain to children and their families. The case of PKU, discussed in the chart above, is a good example. I have worked with adults whose PKU was not detected at birth. They had profound mental retardation and lived in an institutional setting their whole lives. A simple blood test and diet have given many children a better start on life.

But we have to ask ourselves what it means to have a "perfect" baby? In our effort to relieve the burden of suffering caused by severe birth defects, might we open ourselves to the confusion of having to choose which babies are worth saving? Won't we have to ask ourselves which kinds of lives are worth living?

At a conference a few years ago, I met Ann Forts, a woman who refers to her condition as "Up syndrome." She says, "There's nothing 'down' about it." She is a charming, energetic self-advocate who has brought much to the lives of the people who know her. If our tests and treatments could have made her different from what she is, should we have changed her? Remember, I believe all people have gifts. Each person's gifts are of value to all of us.

Right now, we are still years away from a magic fix for most genetic conditions. But we have to start thinking about these issues now. Especially if you are working to support people with disabilities, you must believe that those people are capable of having full, satisfying lives that enrich our communities.

You'll find many people, often the ones who refer to "birth *defects*," who believe developmental disabilities can be eradicated by genetic science. It chills me to think we might jump too quickly on the chance to "cure" everybody and rob ourselves of the diversity and difference that make humanity so enduring. But that's another of my personal prejudices.

A lot of developmental disabilities, though, are not caused by unavoidable genetic accidents. Many children are born with developmental disorders that are caused by things that are easy to prevent. They're caused by mothers using drugs and alcohol when they're pregnant. They're caused by poor nutrition that doesn't allow developing minds to grow. They're caused by abuse that damages children emotionally and physically. They're caused by neglectful parenting that wastes the precious early years of learning. These are social issues we surely need to tackle with all the resources we can bring to bear. But let's go slow on the medical/genetic interventions. What do you think?

PREVENTION—
IT STARTS BEFORE CONCEPTION

Though I have some serious reservations about the current state of genetic research, I still strongly believe every child deserves as good a start in life as possible.

A good start begins before conception. That's right, before. And it's not just the mother's job. There is some research that indicates both the father's sperm and the mother's eggs can be damaged by drugs (including alcohol), radiation, poor nutrition and other environmental factors. Such damage can be prevented. Sexually active people of childbearing age must either take effective steps to prevent conception or maintain the kind of health and well-being that assure a successful pregnancy.

We have much work to do in this area. I was once part of the team evaluating the referral of a four-year-old boy to a group home where I worked. Shortly after the boy was born, his mother, a crack cocaine addict, abandoned him to the care of his grandmother. The grandmother was seeking placement for the little boy. She brought the boy into the conference room in a small wheelchair. He was held upright by straps across the back of the chair. His eyes were slightly crossed and he drooled onto the bib tied around his neck.

We professionals asked the grandmother a series of questions—an assessment—to see if the child would be appropriate for the home we were opening. After many questions about the boy's behavior, the grandmother finally said in frustration, "Let me put it this way—he don't do nothing. Oh, sometimes he can hold his head up." The boy was four years old and would require total care for the rest of his life. And it all could have been prevented!

Some legal advocates are proposing we punish mothers who use drugs and alcohol while they are pregnant. I don't think punishment will work here any more than it does in any other situation. The answer is in motivating people to act responsibly.

As someone who works with people who have developmental disabilities, you can be part of the educational program. If you are of childbearing age, you can take care of yourself. You can tell your friends what you've learned and impress on them the seriousness of what can happen to a developing baby. Education is key.

EARLY INTERVENTION—EACH CHILD NEEDS...

Let's take another look at Ann, the woman with "Up syndrome." When I heard Ann speak, she told of the support she had gotten from her family. I knew that's what had made Ann a confident, poised young woman. Ann had obviously received quality educational programs, along with a stimulating home environment and good medical care. It was these supports, begun shortly after birth, that helped Ann become a contributing member of her community.

Babies with Down syndrome and some other conditions are born with features that tell doctors and parents immediately this child will require special support. For others, it's not so clear at birth. Parents have to observe how the baby develops.

Most children develop in a fairly predictable fashion. Through years of observation, child development specialists have produced lists of "developmental milestones." These are the new things a baby can do at a particular age. For example:

At 1 month, most children:
- Lift head a little when lying on stomach
- Watch objects for a short time
- Make "noise in throat" sounds
- Stay away from annoying sensations such as cloth or blanket on the face

At 6 months, most children:
- Sit with little support
- Respond to a friendly voice with a smile or coo
- Roll from back to stomach
- Turn and look at sounds
- Change object from hand to hand and from hand to mouth

At 12 months, most children:
- Pull themselves to stand and may step with support
- Can nod their head to signal "yes"
- Give love
- Pick things up with thumb and one finger
- Say two or three words

At 18 months, most children:
- Walk (may run a bit)
- Use five to ten words
- Climb up or down one stair
- Pull toys that have wheels
- Mark on paper with crayons
- Understand easy directions

At 2 years, most children:
- Give toys when asked
- Recognize a familiar picture and know if it is upside down
- Kick large ball
- Turn pages in a book (two or three at a time)
- Use two or three words together, such as "more juice"

Notice that each stage says "most children." The developmental milestones are the average time at which an infant picks up new skills. A few months earlier or later is not a problem. But if at the child's first birthday he still can't sit up or roll over, if at his second birthday he can't walk or talk, parents have reason to be concerned.

That concern should lead the parents to have the child evaluated by a child development expert. Many communities have developmental evaluation centers, part of the early intervention movement. These centers are staffed by experts who know that the earlier it is determined that the child needs extra supports, the earlier those supports can be put in place. One study in 1990 looked at children with low birth weights (an indicator of high risk of developmental delays). Those children who received intensive support in the first three years of life achieved significantly higher scores on IQ tests than those children who didn't receive the services. Services offered children from birth to age three are called "early childhood intervention services." A child who receives such support very early in her development is more likely to grow up healthy, strong, and independent.

In the United States, early intervention services were encouraged (through funding) by two sections of the Individuals with Disabilities Education Act (IDEA) of 1986. One section (Part C) provided funding for comprehensive early intervention services for children birth through age two. Another section (Part B), the Preschool Grant Program, offered education services to children ages 3-5. These programs, like IDEA itself (see below) require children to have an Individual Family Support Plan (IFSP) and for services to be delivered in the Least Restrictive Environment (LRE).

IDEA, IFSP, LRE—by now you're probably tearing your hair out in confusion. Not to worry. You don't need to know all the ins and outs of the bureaucracy. Besides, it's changing all the time. New rulings, new interpretations, and new guidelines come out every year. There are professionals whose full-time job is trying to keep up with it all. What's important for you to know is that, just like with ICF-MR, all of these programs offer funding that is dependent on states and local agencies following the rules. The intent is that every child gets a good start on life, to make the best use of whatever gifts he or she was born with. Early recognition of developmental delays and early beginning of support services for children and their families generally goes under the name of "early intervention services."

KEEPING FAMILIES STRONG

Strong families are key to the success of early intervention programs. Children with disabilities present special challenges. They are often irritable, frustrated at their own inability to keep up with the other kids. They are often difficult to toilet train, a milestone most parents are usually thankful for. Some kids, particularly those who have autism, can be withdrawn, not giving Mom and Dad the usual hugs and smiles that help parents get through the tough times.

Parent support groups can make the difference between a family that copes and one that falls apart. Many communities have such groups, often led by experienced professionals who can also help parents get the training and other resources they need, such as babysitters, playgroups and libraries.

Sometimes the thing a family needs most is a break. The other kids grow up, become more independent, spend more time outside the home with their friends and, finally, leave. The child with a disability may require constant attention and support. Respite (RESS-pit) services provide the break.

Sometimes respite is offered through a professional person like yourself coming into the family's home and offering support to the family member with disabilities while the family goes away. Sometimes respite is offered at a facility like a group home. The family brings their son or daughter to the site. Or respite can be offered in the provider's home. Sometimes people who work in residential or vocational support services during the week will support someone in their home on the weekends. Respite services can be key in preventing family burnout; and, where they're well done, they can provide a welcome break for the person with a disability, as well. Remember how Mom and Dad sometimes used to drive you crazy?

THE BIG DECISION—AT HOME OR AWAY

When the resources aren't available, parents may face the most terrible decision of all—whether to place their child in a residential setting away from home. I have talked with such parents, and their stories are wrenching.

The mother of a girl with severe mental retardation told me of how her husband had left her when Nan was born. He couldn't handle the fact that his daughter wasn't "perfect." The now single mother had to work to support Nan and herself. But Nan was a difficult child, and Mom couldn't keep baby sitters. She told me of coming home from work one day to find that the babysitter had fled. Five-year-old Nan

197

had been left alone for several hours. During that time, she had "painted" the entire kitchen with feces. Mom told of sitting on the floor in tears of desperation. The next day, she called the mental health agency to have Nan placed at Colin Anderson Center. It was the hardest thing she ever did, but she felt she had nowhere else to turn.

Some families, frankly, see having a son or daughter with a disability as an unfair burden. The state facility, miles away and already paid for with their tax money, is a place where the child can be dumped, with only a minimum twinge of guilt. Many, many of the people I've worked with in institutional settings have little or no contact with family members, despite the sincere efforts of legions of social workers to keep families intact.

But families value institutional placements for more positive reasons, as well. They may be told, when their child is quite young, by physicians and other trusted professionals, that putting their child in a residential facility is "the only alternative" or "the best thing." Families often see public residential facilities as safe places, where their son or daughter will not be exploited or harassed. They see public facilities as being able to offer the trained staff and specialized programs they are unable to provide at home.

Seldom is the child asked what he wants. Of course, it's common that children do not have the same decision-making rights as adults. But most families prepare children for major change events and pay attention to their reactions.

If a child has a developmental disability, though, things are sometimes done "for their own good" that may have profoundly damaging consequences. I heard of a 12-year-old boy who was afraid to ride in the car because on several occasions, a car ride had actually been a move. While one staff person took him for a ride, the others packed up his stuff and moved it to a new residence. At the end of the ride, the boy was "home" in his new place. Does it surprise you that he was a very disturbed and anxious young man?

We must be careful that we, as professionals, don't violate the bonds of children with their families just because an interdisciplinary team decides it's best. One of the ways I have violated children's rights in the past is with the so-called "transition period." When children moved into group homes I have worked in, we told the parents it would be best if they didn't visit for a couple of weeks. That was supposed to let the child "settle in." That decision was made with terrible consequences for a boy I'll call "Jeremy."

Jeremy was a wild child before he ever moved to the group home. He had torn up his room at home so many times that he slept on a mattress on the floor. He had been moved from one school program to another because his violent tantrums were a danger to all. But when we moved him to the new group home, we really sent him over the edge. Jeremy had no language skills, so there was no way to explain to him what was going on. All he knew was that his parents brought him to a strange house, put his clothes in a new bedroom, then left.

The strangers who now surrounded him were well trained (I trained them) and well-meaning. But Jeremy acted like he had been taken prisoner behind enemy lines. He wouldn't eat. He wouldn't sleep. He ripped up any clothes we tried to put on him. He broke the window in his bedroom, ripped the carpet off the floor, and pulled electrical sockets out of the wall. He screamed and cried day and night. We didn't understand Jeremy. At the time, I thought we were doing a fine job, following "best practice" as we knew it. Looking back, I realize how deeply we had scared and betrayed him.

Regardless of what the team may think of the quality of parenting the child has been getting, regardless of how proud they are of the new opportunity being provided, we must never lose sight of the deep bonds children have with their families. We violate those bonds at everyone's peril.

AVOIDING "PLACEMENT"

In many places, public agencies and private support providers are meeting the challenge of keeping children out of institutional placements. These providers operate on the principal that no one will care for or love a child as well as the child's family. Children who grow up surrounded by loving, committed caretakers become more confident, happier, more independent adults than those raised by an ever-changing line-up of paid staff.

If you work in a program that provides supports for children with disabilities, remember that it is your job to do *with* rather than do *for*. You can work *with* families to provide the additional support they need rather than raising their child *for* them. As a trained professional, you can show parents ways of dealing with challenging behavior, ways of teaching new skills, and ways of building supportive relationships that can make the difference between a child who stays home and one who moves to an institutional placement.

GROWING UP; BREAKING AWAY

One of the most important tasks families may need help with is allowing their child with disabilities to grow into an adult. Though I have said I agree with the notion that children's needs are best served by loving families, I have to warn you about something that often happens in such families. When a child is always dependent on his parents, he may lose the opportunity to grow up. The whole family may see him as "our baby."

These attitudes are usually well motivated. Parents may want to protect their adult son or daughter from embarrassment or exploitation. Or they may value the company they provide. Mom and Dad can avoid the "empty nest" syndrome by keeping one of the children at home and dependent on them. All the other kids grew up and left, but not "my baby."

When parents don't let their children grow up there can be conflict between the generations. Suddenly "my baby" doesn't want to be "Johnny" any more. He would rather be called "John." And he wants a real job, not just the safe place at the workshop his parents got for him. And he wants to have his girlfriend over to spend the night. As John's support person, you want to empower him to be all he can be. But you run head on into Mom and Dad.

The best approach is to be diplomatic and work on building relationships. You cannot advocate effectively by getting in people's faces. Mom and Dad have probably had it up to here with well-meaning professionals who've given advice (often conflicting) on how they ought to raise their son. They're not interested in what your Vocational Assessment shows about John's work skills. They've heard all that assessment jargon many times before. What you have to do is win their trust. You can show them you understand how scary it is to think of John out in the big, bad world. And you can help John show Mom and Dad some small successes that, though risky, have paid off. One step at a time.

Sheila was one of the women we worked with at Access, Inc. She wanted to get a job, but her mother, who she lived with, was absolutely against it. So Sheila's community coach started building bridges with Mom. At the end of each day, when she brought Sheila home, the coach would chat with Mom. They shared life experiences. They shared little successes. Gradually, the coach won Mom's trust.

One day the coach felt confident enough to help Sheila approach her Mom about a job. They already had the job lined up. The coach would be with Sheila every day. The employer had already successfully hired other people with disabilities. Mom said, "OK, as long as you'll be with her. I'll let her try it."

Sheila's new job was a turning point in her life. A year later, she was saving money for her own apartment...with Mom's support. Sometimes the most important thing a support person can do is "take what you can get closest to what you want."

Caring for a family member with developmental disabilities is difficult. When parents have chosen to keep guardianship of their son or daughter, the family plan for "what happens when Mom and Dad die" is often to transfer guardianship to a brother or sister. That sibling may have his or her own family responsibilities and agree to take charge of the disabled brother or sister, while still resenting having to.

Good future planning, making sure that all stakeholders are heard, can help families come up with alternatives. The choice is seldom "move in with me or go to an institution." Many innovative programs offer a range of supports which allow family relationships to remain intact and give people with disabilities the opportunity to have meaningful lives of their own.

"FREE, APPROPRIATE EDUCATION"

If you work with adults who have developmental disabilities, you can piece together your own history of how we in the United States have changed our approach to support services. If the person you work with turned 18 before 1975, he probably never went to public school. If he did start school, he probably "flunked out" in the early grades. He was sent home, the school telling his parents, "We can't do anything with him."

If you work with someone who was a child in 1975, she may have benefited from a law that caused sweeping changes. The Education of all Handicapped Children Act (PL94-142) was passed in 1975. In 1997, the law was amended and now goes under the name of IDEA (Individuals with Disabilities Education Act). Both versions of the law set some clear benchmarks for public education of children with a variety of disabilities.

The law says every child in the United States is entitled to a free, appropriate public education, regardless of the child's handicapping condition. Every local education agency (LEA) is responsible for seeing that every child who has a disability will have an Individualized Education Plan (IEP) and will be educated in the "least restrictive environment" (our old friend LRE).

What that means in simpler terms is that a local school system can no longer tell the parents of a child with a disability that they have no program for that child. It means that each school district has to have annual planning sessions that include the child, the child's parents, and any other advocate or professional person the family wants to have present. It means the family gets to decide what is appropriate for their child. It means that the child must be educated in an environment that is as close as possible to that enjoyed by other children of the same age and in the same community. It means the parents are not required to pay for extra services their child needs. And it means the child is entitled to these educational services until the end of the school year in which she turns 21.

That's a lot of requirements. Some school systems do a great job. Children attend class in regular classrooms along with typical kids (called "mainstreaming"). Parents are active participants in IEP sessions. And there is a wide range of specialized services available as needed.

As you can imagine, though, some school systems have been dragged kicking and screaming into the world of integrated special education. I once attended an evening meeting that was called by the local school district for the purpose of informing parents why their children were being moved from a self-contained class at an elementary school to a self-contained class at a high school. The reason for the move was that it seemed more "age appropriate" for the kids who were fourteen years old and older to be at the school for older kids. The parents were irate because it meant bussing their kids across the county.

I went to the meeting because several of the children in the class lived in a group home I was working with. I also thought the bureaucrats were missing the point—that the kids should go to the high school because they were high school age and should have an opportunity to mix with their age peers. The parents, on the other hand, were worried that age peer mixing would be a bad thing. They pointed out that since kids with disabilities and typical kids had been educated in separate schools all along, the typical kids had no idea of what the other kids were about. They were worried that their kids, who had grown up in a sheltered, segregated school system, would be harassed, laughed at or exploited. They were worried that their kids would spend hours on the bus. They felt their rights were being violated.

The school officials got defensive and even lied a time or two. At one point, a father raised his hand to speak. He had a little book open in his lap. It was the Parent Handbook every school district is required to give parents of students with disabilities. It outlines their rights under the law. The man said, "It says here that my daughter should be educated in the same environment as she would if she didn't have a handicap. Well, I live in the eastern end of the county, and that would be East High School, not being bussed all the way over to West." There was a round of applause from the other parents. The Special Education Coordinator then told the crowd that in fact the law does not require them to make special services available at every school. The services for the man's daughter were available...at West High School.

I had to pipe up. I told the parents the law puts them in the driver's seat. If they don't agree with the program that's proposed for their child, they don't sign the IEP. The school system would then be out of compliance with the law and would collect no special education funds for that child until the parent signs. If the school resists, there is a formal appeal process. I told them I had seen many cases where parents won their appeals and many more where the school system offered what they wanted before it got to a formal appeal. I received a round of applause from the parents...and hostile glares from the school officials.

A NEW IDEA

When the old special education law was amended in 1997 to become IDEA, it made some much needed changes in the way education services are delivered to children with special needs. Some of the most important changes are:

- Parents are now included in groups making eligibility and placement decisions about children with disabilities.
- Schools must send parents regular progress reports on their child.
- Regular classroom teachers must be included in IEP meetings, and the IEP must address what kinds of supports are needed for the child to be successful in a regular classroom.
- States must gather data to show that they are not discriminating against people from minority groups or who have limited English speaking ability.
- Challenging behavior that is in some way part of a child's disability must be dealt with as an educational issue in the IEP. Children entitled to special education services can be expelled only for bringing weapons and drugs to the classroom. Even then, their needed supports must continue in a non-school setting.

That last issue continues to cause a lot of conflict. Many schools, frustrated by a rising tide of student violence, have adopted "zero tolerance" policies. Under these policies, any student who commits an aggressive act is suspended from school or kicked out altogether. But "zero tolerance" and good special education practice sometimes conflict.

Do you remember Eddie from Chapter 7? He was the young man who was learning to go to his "safe haven" when he was upset, instead of hitting people. As I said in the earlier story, Eddie was making some progress.

Then one day I got called to a meeting with the principal of Eddie's school. It seems Eddie had yelled at his teacher and pulled his fist back as if he was going to hit her. He didn't actually swing at her, but the mere threat violated the school's zero tolerance policy. They were going to kick Eddie out of school, because "it isn't fair to let one child get away with it." I was livid and almost needed to be restrained myself. I asked the principal how he could kick Eddie out of school for a behavior that his IEP said he was learning to deal with. The principal gave in a little. He said Eddie could stay for now but that he would be kicked out if it happened "one more time." I left the school frustrated at the stupidity of bureaucracy, but I had bought Eddie a little more time to learn to get his act together.

You too can be an advocate for children you work with. You don't have to know all the details of all the bureaucratic rules and procedures. But you do need to know enough to help families stand up for the rights they are guaranteed by law. You need to know that the IEP process puts the family in the driver's seat. They don't have to follow instructions when the school calls and says they should "swing by the office sometime and sign your child's IEP." They don't have to accept what the school system says is "all we have."

You need to know that "least restrictive environment" means mainstreaming, unless the school can prove the child's needs can only be met in a segregated placement. Not only does mainstreaming prepare children with disabilities for a life in the rest of the world, but it also educates typical kids about diversity. These kids are the adult citizens of tomorrow. If they go to school with kids who have different gifts and gaps from the usual, they may become business owners who hire people with disabilities and neighbors who welcome their old classmates to the neighborhood.

And you need to know that children must receive services (addressing the ever-changing goals of the IEP) until they are 21. Transitional services, helping a young person move from school into the world of work, must begin when the child reaches the age of 14. Those services must prepare young people to be employed, to have meaningful relationships, and to live as independently in their communities as possible. The School-to-Work Opportunities Act (STWO) of 1994 emphasized preparation for work for all students who have had difficulties in adult life due to race, gender, and disabilities.

Armed with those tools, you can be an effective advocate for effective educational services.

AGING WITH A DISABILITY

When people reach adulthood and finish school, they usually look forward to getting a job and getting their own home. We'll deal with those important life stages in the next chapter. For now, we'll move on to the last stage of the lifecycle—aging.

You've probably heard a lot about "the graying of America." People are living longer, and those who were born during the post-war baby boom are entering their 50's.

People with disabilities are also living longer, though not as long as the general population. In the general population, women now live to around age 79 and men usually live to around age 73. A recent study found that among people with developmental disabilities age 40 and older without Down syndrome, the average age of death was 67 for women and 63 for men. For people age 40 and older with Down syndrome, the average age of death was 57 for women and 54 for men.

Improved health care services and better living conditions have meant that people who once would have faced an early death are now living into their "golden years." It is estimated that between 200,000 and 500,000 people in the United States over the age of 60 have some form of developmental disability. Some of these people live at home with elderly parents or other family caregivers. Others live in small community programs or foster care. But over half of all people with mental retardation over the age of 62 who live in residential placements live in nursing homes.

If these elders who have disabilities are in "training programs" they continue to be subjected to the usual silliness. I knew one 62-year-old man who was being trained to write his name. I wondered how many thousands of hours of his life had been wasted on this "necessary" task that he was obviously unable to accomplish. He also had to go to the sheltered workshop every day because that was the only "day placement" available. He was depressed and lonely.

Instead of "supported employment," elders with disabilities need the opportunity for "supported retirement." Most people with disabilities who are in their 60's now lived many years in large institutional places. They were probably abused at one time or another. They were almost certainly neglected. I think they need a break. Not to sit in the hall in wheelchair all day; that's not what I'm suggesting. They need a break in the usual requirements, a chance to hang out with their buds at the local senior center or linger over a cup of coffee at McDonald's.

HEALTHY AGING

Many people think that people with mental retardation experience more serious health problems as they age than people without disabilities. On the whole, that's not necessarily true. But some studies show that the age-related health needs of people with disabilities are underreported and undertreated. There are some increased risks you should know about if you work with an older person with disabilities.

For instance, people with Down syndrome seem to begin the aging process earlier than their peers without disabilities, which causes the shorter life expectancy cited above. Adults with Down syndrome are also at increased risk for Alzheimer's disease. Whereas approximately six percent of the general population will develop the disease, the figure is about 25 percent for people with Down syndrome.

People with cerebral palsy may be at greater risk for developing a number of bone, muscle, and joint-related diseases as they age, such as scoliosis (abnormal curvature of the spine) and spinal stenosis (neurological problems associated with narrowing of the spinal canal).

Women with developmental disabilities may be at greater risk for osteoporosis and related bone fractures due to amenorrhea (the absence of periods), earlier menopause, the use of certain medications (anticonvulsants, excessive thyroid hormones, steroids), and because they are more likely to be inactive or experience falls.

Women with developmental disabilities often have not received information about the nature of menstrual periods and menopause. Therefore, it is important to inform women about menopause and to arrange for periodic evaluations by a health care professional with expertise in women's health.

As people get older, their vision and hearing usually get worse. A person who can't tell you what's happening with her may appear withdrawn or irritable. Thorough vision and hearing evaluations can restore some of their old ability, so they enjoy favorite activities again.

You can help people with disabilities live longer and happier lives by:

- Watching for behavioral changes that may indicate an underlying health problem, especially for people who have communication difficulties

- Ensuring access to appropriate health information and to health professionals who are experienced in diagnosing and treating age-related health problems

- Seeing that older women receive regular screenings and examinations for early detection of breast, ovarian and uterine cancer, especially if they are sexually active or postmenopausal

- Seeing that older men have regular screenings and examinations for prostate problems and colorectal cancer

- Helping people understand the changes that are happening in their bodies as they age

PLANNING AND SUPPORT

Aging doesn't have to be a time of sickness and inactivity. Some people may want to continue working. This will be especially true if the person you're working with has only recently found his first job. The job may be his primary contact with the larger community, and it's probably where his friends are.

Some people want to travel, while others want to spend more time at home. Others may want to spend time with age peers at a senior center. Norman, the 65-year-old man who agreed to cut down on his cigarettes (Chapter 11), was nominated for the "Volunteer of the Year" award by the Retired Senior Volunteers Program (RSVP) because of his work delivering Meals on Wheels.

Person-centered planning is critical in helping these people make choices about how they would like to live out the remaining part of their lives. Many older people with disabilities, who have spent years in institutional environments, have not had the opportunity to make choices or develop plans. Or they may have lived most of their lives at home as "the baby" and know very little about what older adults do. You will need to be patient and supportive.

Older people in general start remembering more about the long past and forgetting what happened yesterday. Talking with them about what their lives have been like, helping them make a scrapbook of photos and mementos from significant events, may help them get perspective on their lives.

A GOOD DEATH

Finally, there is the matter of dying. It is a subject that is scary and confusing to most of us. Yet we all have to think about it eventually. Either we have to face our own death or that of a close loved one.

Decisions have to be made about what kinds of medical interventions a person wants at the end of life. Decisions have to be made about funerals and burial. These are tough decisions for all of us. Think how much harder it is for someone who has a limited understanding of these things. Families will need a lot of support to help their family member make these end-of-life decisions.

The common approach is to think, "Oh, well; she doesn't understand about death, so we just won't talk about it." Sometimes that's not good enough. I once had to take a 15-year-old girl who had moderate mental retardation to the funeral of her father. The casket was open, according to the family's wish. I asked Karen if she would like to look. She said yes, she was excited about seeing her Daddy. We walked up to the open casket, and Karen started calling, "Daddy, Daddy," while patting on his chest as if he would wake up. She then turned to me and said seriously, as if she had just discovered the fact, "James, I think my Daddy's dead." Never underestimate what people with disabilities understand.

Birth, childhood, school days, and a graceful old age—these are stages in real life in the real world. You will need to understand the particular needs of people with disabilities at all stages, as you help them share that real life with us.

Chapter 13

A HOME AND A JOB IN THE REAL WORLD

I was 19 years old when I got my first apartment. I had been living in the dorm at college, and my roommate and I decided it was time to move off campus. We found a three room apartment that was the lower part of an old house. The rent was $60 a month. The place was pretty run down, but we rolled up our sleeves and gave it a good cleaning (we found a dead cat in the cupboard under the kitchen sink). We put Indian print bedspreads over the windows, hung posters on the wall (it was the '60's), and invited our friends over for a housewarming party. It was great. The toilet was constantly backing up, the windows leaked snow in the wintertime, and the cockroaches were fulltime pets. But it was my own place. I could decide when to come and go, who to allow in and who to keep out, what to eat, what music to listen to. My parents thought it was a dump, but I thought of it as home.

Having our own home is a life goal of most of us. It's part of growing up. We find out who we are as we set up housekeeping and become responsible adults. Home is where we are most truly ourselves.

That's not always the case for people with disabilities. Their need for supports sometimes limits their options to living in the places where the supports are provided. That usually means either living at home with Mom and Dad or moving to a residential facility. Residential facilities generally come in two flavors—large and small.

FACILITIES LARGE AND SMALL

Big state-run residential facilities usually serve a large geographical catchment area, so they are often far away from a person's family, friends and familiar places. Moving to a place like that, as we have seen, is often the first step in segregation.

The living areas of large facilities, often called "cottages" or "lodges," are generally organized according to the nature of the person's disability. All of the people who require extra medical services, for instance, often live in an area close to the hospital. People with behavior challenges are often placed in a "high control" unit where staff are trained and equipped to deal with aggressive outbursts. The placements are based on similar needs, rather than on similar interests. Everyone living together has the same gaps. There is no opportunity to spend time with people whose gifts might help a person overcome his gaps. This type of segregation based on need keeps people from establishing natural supports and thus keeps them dependent on the system.

Small residential facilities, usually called "group homes," are more often located in communities where other people live. Group home sizes generally range from ten people to two people. The people who operate group homes (I've been one) try to remember to refer to them as the "home" of the people who live there. But they are almost always licensed facilities that have to follow regulatory requirements set down by various government agencies.

If I operate a licensed residential facility, I am responsible to see that it is safe and clean. I hire the people who work there, and I am responsible for their performance. I choose who lives in the home, usually from a list of referrals made by the local governing body. In short, it's *my* home, no matter how hard I try to make it appear otherwise.

A HOME OF ONE'S OWN

A home of one's own is a new flavor on the menu of residential opportunities for people with disabilities. How does one's own home look different from what I've just described? I think there are two characteristics that are important:
- who controls the front door, and
- how integrated the residence is with the rest of the neighborhood.

Who controls the front door is a critical question. I used to think it was a question of people having a key to where they live. I worked hard to be sure everyone had a key, even those people the house staff said were unable to use theirs. It was largely a symbolic gesture. You don't really control the front door of your home unless you control who else has a key to your house. Even when the people who lived there had keys to the group homes I worked at, there were still lots of other people who came and went as they pleased. I have never worked in a group home where the people who lived there chose the house, chose who else lived in the house, and chose who worked in the house. Would you think you had a home of your own if you were placed at a house you'd never seen before? Would you think it was your home if you had five roommates you'd never met before? And what about all these strangers coming in and out, people who think of the place not as your home but as their workplace?

Sometimes we try to cover all the negative issues of group home placement by pretending the residents and staff are a "family." But how many families do you know of that are made up of six unrelated "kids" and a dozen rotating "moms and dads?"

The problem with the family model is that there is no such thing as a "typical" family. My family life was different from yours. We baked a ham for Easter, while your family didn't eat pork. We walked around in our underwear; your Mom sent you to your room. My northern European family spoke softly in the house, while your Italian one spoke with loud voices and lots of hands.

We all grow up with certain expectations about the way life ought to be—and that includes people with disabilities. When we control the front door to a home of our own we get to set the standard for what our life should be like. We get to go to bed and get up when we please. We get to be messy or neat. We get to put out the welcome mat or keep the door locked tight against strangers.

Then there's the issue of integration with the neighborhood. You may recall that integration's opposite, segregation, was one of the primary characteristics of the institutional mindset. Realizing that this was a problem in the large, state-run facilities, the deinstitutionalization movement sought to move people "into the community."

Thousands of small residences were built or renovated, and people were moved out of the big, centralized places. But these new homes often stayed isolated from the rest of the neighborhood. Why was that? Because people in the neighborhood are not fooled. They know the place is not a home like theirs. They think of it more as a business that has been thrust into the middle of their neighborhood. Staff are coming and going at all hours of the day or night (and parking all up and down the block when there's a staff meeting). And how can you get to know six new neighbors and their six new staff all at once? Do you bring over a dozen casseroles?

Of course, getting to know the neighbors when you move into a new place is not only a problem for people with disabilities. I lived in my last residence for three years. I knew the last names of two families (from their mailboxes) and maybe half a dozen people by their first names. My neighbors were not my friends. And that's not uncommon. A recent study by Robert Putnam at Harvard University showed community connectedness is down for all groups. He found that there are 60% fewer club meetings, 60% fewer picnics, and fewer community bowling leagues, than a couple of decades ago. Many of us now choose to live in a smaller social world that revolves around a few close friends, family, and co-workers.

But people with disabilities have had isolation forced on them. Many people who have lived in institutional settings are desperately seeking a life filled with friends, neighbors and co-workers. They want to learn how to act in the real world, and they want the rewards and relationships of being included in everyday life. We do these people a disservice if we "place" groups of them into neighborhoods in a way that makes the potential neighbors see them as an alien invasion force.

When people choose their own neighborhood, they are likely to choose a setting in which they feel comfortable. They will choose a place where they feel free to be who they truly are. It will be a place where the rhythms and habits of life are like those they grew up in.

I believe sometime in the not too distant future we will see living in a group residence as an unacceptable limitation of a person's right to choose where and with whom he lives. And maybe "residential placements" will be replaced by more natural living options that still provide needed supports.

WHAT OPTIONS ARE AVAILABLE NOW?

OPEN RESIDENCES

As long as the current system of funding for residential services requires groups of people to live in licensed facilities we'll have to do the best we can with what we've got. We can at least make those facilities into what I call "open residences." If you work in one of those places, I suggest you:

- **Offer people a choice of homes.** Asking someone whether he wants to live in the Oak Group Home or the Maple Group Home is not the same as helping him look through the classifieds like my college roommate and I did. But at least it's the beginning of a choice. A person who is moving either from a large facility or from their parents' home, should have a chance to see a couple of different houses, meet the other residents and staff (supper is a good time) and choose which she feels more comfortable in. Remember, if she can't speak, you'll have to pay close attention to her reaction to the places. She'll let you know which she prefers.

- **Offer people a choice of housemates.** There are a lot of people I wouldn't want to live with. And there's only one person I want to share a bedroom with. Be careful you don't put incompatible people together and then put them on behavior training programs to teach them to get along. Unrelated people do often share housing space, either for company or to help pay the bills. But even when someone advertises for a roommate, he reserves the right to ask that person to leave if things don't work out.

    People who have lived a long time in the disabilities support system usually know the others in their area. They've had to live together in the large facilities or work together in sheltered employment. They often have a history. Yet I've seen case managers ignore the fact that John and Jerry hate each other and have fought every place they've been. Likewise, professionals often ignore people's stated preferences. If Cindy says she'd like to have Louis as her roommate because he's her best friend, what are you going to do?

- **Offer people a choice of support staff.** I heard about an agency that decided to take this one seriously. They told the four men living together in one of the group homes that they could choose their own staff. The first thing the men did was fire the current staff.

Imagine if you had a disabling accident and needed someone to come into your home to help you with things. Wouldn't you demand the right to choose who that person is and to get rid of someone you feel treats you badly in any way? I feel strongly that no support staff should be hired until they've met and been approved by the people they're going to support.

- **Remember that this is their home—you're only the hired help.** When I've visited the group homes I've been associated with, I always rang the doorbell. Sometimes the staff would look out the window, and I could hear them saying, "It's James; what's he doing?" Then one of the staff would open the door, and I'd say, "Oh, I'm sorry; I must have the wrong house. I was looking for David." My co-worker would look at me as if to say, "James, what's wrong with you?" It was a feeble symbolic gesture, to be sure, but I wanted to remind myself, as well as the others, that if this was the home of the people who lived there, they needed to control the front door. They also need to control the telephone, the grocery list and the schedule.

  We've talked a lot about the kinds of choices adults who live in their own homes get to make. One way to honor those choices in group living environments is to make sure the staff make NO decisions about the place. No, you can't decorate the house for Halloween. No, you can't decide on the smoking policy. No, you can't decide what to watch on TV, which night to go to the mall, or whether it's time to replace the living room sofa. All of those decisions, and many more, should be made by the people who live in the house. They may need support and assistance making those decisions, for sure. But all staff have to remember their place. This is not your home.

  One of the most important parts of my home being my home is that it's private. I can act and dress in ways here that I don't do in public. People who have to live in group residences should have the same privilege. People should be able to let their hair down at home and be their private selves.

- **Become a bridge to the neighborhood.** Then become invisible. If you don't want the neighbors to think of the group home as an illegally operated neighborhood business, don't act like it's your job site. You should feel privileged to be allowed to come into a person's home to support her in her life. Just like any other training or support program, you need to fade into the background and let the person you support live his life—with his neighbors, friends and co-workers.

IN-HOME SUPPORTS/SUPPORTED LIVING

As we saw in Chapter 4, support services for people with disabilities are moving toward self-determination. In residential services, all the decisions I talked about above should be made by the person with disabilities and his family.

The first step is for people not to have to move to a residential facility to get the supports they need. Those supports should be provided wherever the person who needs them chooses to live. This model is usually referred to as "in-home supports" or "supported living." In-home supports can be provided either in the person's parent's home if they choose to stay there or in some other residence of their choosing.

In the United States, the issue of in-home supports is being addressed by a piece of legislation called the Medicaid Community Attendant Services and Supports Act. This bill is also known by its acronym, MiCASSA, which is pronounced like "mi casa," Spanish for "my house." Though at the time of the writing of this book MiCASSA is still languishing in committee, many advocacy groups are supporting its passage. The introduction to the bill lists some "findings" that are relevant to our discussion of supported living opportunities:

- "While many people with disabilities want to receive supports in their own homes and communities, 75% of Medicaid funds are expended in nursing homes and ICFs/MR," where you have to move in to receive services.
- "Decisions regarding…services and supports are too often influenced by what is reimbursable…" Support provider agencies have to get paid. They naturally provide the services they can get paid for.
- "Long-term services and supports provided under the Medicaid program must meet the evolving…needs and preferences…for living within one's own home or living with one's own family and becoming productive members of the community."
- "The goals of the Nation" should include:
    a) a meaningful choice of receiving long-term services and supports in the most integrated setting appropriate;

b) the greatest possible control over the services received;
c) quality services that maximize functioning in home and community.

In-home supports have several advantages over residential facilities:

- **It's clear whose home it is.** When you are an in-home support worker, you go to the person's home to work for her. Don't you think you'll remember to ring the doorbell and be invited in?
- **The person receiving supports can live the style of life he's most comfortable with.** That includes when to go to bed and when to get up, what to eat, what to wear, even which room to put the TV set in.
- **A lot of challenging behavior disappears.** As we discussed earlier, a lot of the challenging behavior I've seen in people with disabilities comes from the environment they live in rather than from the disability. A person receiving in-home supports will no longer engage in power struggles with staff. They're her staff; if she doesn't like them, she fires them. There will be no struggle for getting the limited amount of attention available. Each person can contract for however much attention he thinks he needs (and for privacy when he wants people out of his life). We won't expect people who have a hard time getting along with others to live with other people who have the same issues.
- **In-home supports are generally less expensive.** When people are placed into "beds" in residential facilities, they get a whole package of services, some of which they may not need. By offering only the supports the person needs, an amount which should decrease as the person learns to live more independently, the total amount of money spent is no more than current levels.

HOW DO I DO IT?

If you are providing in-home supports or supported living, what exactly do you do? It's a good question, because the job of in-home assistant is different from that of being part of the staff of a residential facility.

First of all, as an in-home support worker, you may be working on your own. This is sometimes referred to as "one-to-one." We used this model at Access, Inc. and we used the term "Community Coach" for support worker. I thought that term conveyed the idea that the support person was a helper, supporter and encourager rather than a trainer and controller. And the "community" part meant that the support worker's job took place in an environment that was free of the boundaries we usually put up between inside and outside the facility.

Just because your job isn't limited to training doesn't mean you won't be helping the person you support learn new skills. You will. But you will be sure they are skills that person thinks he needs to learn. And you will be teaching those skills through participation (informal learning) and in the environment in which they're practiced. Some of the important things people in supported living situations may want to learn include:

- **Personal safety training**—what to do in case of a fire or break-in; how to deal with strangers or harassment from neighbors; how to get assistance when needed; how to safely deal with hazardous substances. Sometimes this involves helping a person set up alarm systems or other supportive technology that is both more effective and less expensive than having a staff person always present.
- **Personal hygiene and health**—how to keep clean and avoid infectious illness; what to do if she's sick or injured; how to take medication.
- **Nutrition and food preparation**—your local health department probably has nutrition pyramid charts. They may even have cooking classes.
- **Social roles and safe sex**—we've talked about this one before. It's a lot easier if you can help the person learn what he needs in the privacy of his own home. And you won't have to fight the group home rules that say he can't have his girlfriend over for dinner.

The most important point about training in a supported living environment is that it is not for the purpose of being "cured" or of getting enough skills so the person becomes "ready" to go somewhere else. Supported living is real life in the real world, right now. It doesn't require people to be someone other than who they actually are.

NATURAL SUPPORTS

Remember in Chapter 6 where we said people with disabilities don't have to be Independent, any more than the rest of us do? Instead of Independence, we are going to go for "Interdependence," where everyone has a network of "natural supports" they can rely on. Nowhere is that more important than in residential support services. One of your jobs as a support provider is to help the person you're supporting locate and set up natural supports

Remember that natural supports are supports that are naturally present in all people's lives. Some examples include: a friend who helps paint your house, a neighbor who picks up your mail when you're out of town, a co-worker who picks up your paycheck when you're sick, the family member who introduces you to a potential new employer.

Maybe you haven't recognized the natural supports in your life because we tend not to call them that. We're more likely to think of our support network as our "community." Inclusion activist Judith Snow defines community as "a series of partnerships that unlock the potential of each of the participants." A person with disabilities who is isolated from the mainstream of society has only limited opportunity to form such mutually unlocking partnerships. But out in the real world, you and the person you support can open doors, hearts and minds.

A community isn't a place you can move to. Your community is the web of supportive relationships (natural supports) you build around yourself. Developing this network of supports is one of the first things you do when you move to a new place, and it should be one of the first things you help the person you support do. You could call what you do "community support outreach." Get out and meet the neighbors and the local merchants. Learn the bus routes and the emergency hot line phone numbers. It's OK for someone to need help with things—we all do. But everyone needs to know where to turn, and you can help with that.

HOME OWNERSHIP

When it comes to living "on our own," the greatest dream we all have is to own our own home. This is a possible dream for people with disabilities, as well. It's probably not the first step for someone who has never lived on his own. That would probably be to rent a place, just as it is with everyone else. But home ownership is something everyone can dream about—and plan for.

If the person you support is interested in owning her own home, you should check out the National Home of Your Own Alliance (NHYO). It was established in 1993 for the purpose of helping people with disabilities own their own homes. They have a very informative website at www.alliance.unh.edu. One of the links from that site takes you to a guide, produced with Fannie Mae, called *A Home of Your Own Guide*.

The guide:
...walks prospective home owners through the complex process of buying a home, from the initial decision to make the purchase, through the steps for acquiring a mortgage, and finally, to life as a homeowner. The new guide introduces a 'person centered approach' to homeownership, which places people with disabilities at the center of the decision-making process on issues affecting their personal lives and living situations.

Cool, eh?

Another route to home ownership for people with disabilities could be Habitat for Humanity. I've long had a dream of people we support volunteering on Habitat projects until, finally, it's their turn to get the keys to their new home.

All of these visions of living on one's own give people more of an opportunity to live a real life in the real world. But they also include one of the realties of life for all of us. You have to pay your bills. And if you're going to pay your bills, you have to have a job.

THE OPPORTUNITY TO WORK

Even back in the 1970's people were talking about work opportunities for people with disabilities. At Colin Anderson Center we had a nursery program where selected residents could grow plants that were then sold for money to support the program. Working at the nursery was very popular, and there was always a waiting list to get in.

At the same time, on the far end of the facility's campus there were the ruins of a dairy farm and sawmill that had been run years before by the people who lived at the center. Work had once been a part of everyone's daily routine. The farm produced the food that everyone ate, and the sawmill produced the lumber that built the buildings.

The only problem was that the residents who worked in these places were not paid for their labor. Instead, working was considered part of earning their keep. When rights advocates made the case that this was exploitative, the institutional farms and factories all shut down. People stayed on their wards and languished in day rooms—or got on the waiting list to work at the nursery.

Work is a dignified part of real life in the real world. Though we all work because we have to support ourselves, most of us expect to get more than money from our jobs. Doing good work gives us a feeling of accomplishment. It is part of who we are. When we meet someone new, one of the first questions we ask is, "What do you do?" And work is where we meet people, people who sometimes become friends.

THE SATISFACTIONS OF WORK

Money, personal satisfaction, relationships—these are some of the rewards of having a meaningful job. Unfortunately, they are rewards that are often denied people with disabilities.

From time to time, studies are done on the economic status of people with disabilities. They always show that poverty and disability are usually found together, at least in the United States. That's because most people with disabilities are unemployed or underemployed.

I mentioned earlier that sheltered workshops can get waivers from the Department of Labor that allow them to pay less than minimum wage. Much of the work is paid by the piece, based on the rate of work of a non-disabled worker. For example, if a regular worker can make 100 widgets per hour and the minimum wage is $5.50 per hour, the piece rate is five and a half cents per widget. If Harry is put to work at a table with other people like him, and he is distracted by watching staff put his co-workers in time out, he may have a day where he makes 10 widgets all day. That's $.55 for a day's work! If the workshop doesn't have any contracts to work on, Harry might spend his day on "work adjustment activities" and make no money at all. At this rate, it's going to be a long time before he can save enough money to buy something he wants.

The second reward of work, personal satisfaction, is one that can be found in sheltered environments. I have toured many of these places and have often been struck by how proud many of the workers are of the work they produce. They work hard, show up regularly, and seem to enjoy simple repetitive tasks. They are glad to tell people in their community that they work every day. When people ask where they work, they proudly say "Allied Exceptional Industries." Everyone smiles and nods their heads, knowing that AEI is where "the handicapped" work, supported by community donations from the United Way campaign.

I played that game for many years, proud of myself for the "opportunity" I was offering people who would otherwise be sitting at home. But that was before I discovered the value of supported employment, a real job in the real world. Once I got my head out of the workshop box I saw that the pride people with disabilities had in their work, the reliability with which they tackled tasks, were skills that were needed in real jobs. And I found that the satisfaction of having a real job was of a different order of magnitude from being proud of having a place at the workshop.

REAL JOBS IN THE REAL WORLD

When we started Access, Inc. we decided everyone who received our services who wanted a job should have a job—a real job. I was not prepared for the boost in self-esteem those people experienced. One man, who worked as a grounds maintenance man at the Hampton Inn, was so proud of his uniform with "Terry" embroidered on the pocket that he wanted to wear it all the time. A man with a job is "somebody."

Hazel worked as a housekeeper at the Holiday Inn. Though she was in her 30's, it was the first real job she'd had in her life. As a Holiday Inn employee, she had an identification card that entitled her to stay at any Holiday Inn in the country for $15 a night. Her job coach said, "I've been trying to get Hazel to plan a time for her and me to go to the beach." Hazel just smiled and said, "No, first I'm gonna take my Mama somewhere." Hazel was an employed person, someone with something to offer.

While we're on the subject of job satisfaction, I need to address "The Four F's." These refer to the categories of jobs people with disabilities often get: Food (which includes fast food restaurants), Filth (cleaning of any kind), Filing (doing repetitive work in offices or mail rooms) and Flowers (working in nurseries, landscaping, lawn care). Often advocates put these categories down, saying they are demeaning and reflect the second class status of people with disabilities. I strongly disagree. I think jobs in the Four F's categories are the kinds of entry level jobs that anyone without work experience or education would do. I certainly did those kinds of jobs while I was going to school. As long as the person is working at a real job that needs to be done, a job that she chose from among various possibilities and that an employer is willing to pay at least minimum wage for, there's nothing demeaning about it. The most demeaning condition is to have no job at all or to be stuck in a "pre-vocational" placement. Too often, "pre-" means "never."

The third advantage of working is the opportunity to build relationships. That's why I'm so down on sheltered employment of any kind. It is segregated and doesn't allow people with disabilities to form meaningful relationships with co-workers who have different gifts from theirs. I don't like the "enclave" model where people with disabilities work in a segregated group within a larger business. I don't like the "mobile crew" model (often used in cleaning or lawn care), where a group of people with disabilities moves from job to job with a more able supervisor. It's not that there is anything "wrong" with these kinds of jobs. It's just that integration in the community is so important for people who've been left out.

A job is often the key that opens the door to acceptance and understanding. Shortly after we started the Access services, I got a call from the housekeeping supervisor at the Holiday Inn where several of our people were working. She just wanted to tell me how glad she was to have the workers we had sent there. She told me how her veteran workers were excited about the upcoming staff Christmas party so their families could have a chance to meet Hazel and the others. And she told me the people with disabilities who were working there had had a positive impact on everyone's work. "My girls," she confided, "sometimes have a bad attitude about this work. They think it's just a crummy job. But they see people who are glad of the opportunity and are proud of their work, and they seem to perk up a bit." Integrated employment is good for everyone.

SUPPORTED EMPLOYMENT

As you can see, I have strong opinions about people with disabilities working. Fortunately, my prejudice in favor of real jobs in the real world is not just a cranky minority view. It's the wave of the future, though it's been a long time coming. In the United States the Rehabilitation Act of 1973 (and amended in 1992) established the concept of "supported employment" as a category of vocational assistance. The Act defined supported employment as:

- competitive work
- in integrated settings
- for persons with the most severe disabilities for whom competitive employment has not occurred or has been interrupted
- who need intensive support services or extended services

"Competitive" means you have to compete for the job in the open job market. It's not a made-up job that's just for people with disabilities.

"Integrated settings" means people with disabilities work alongside co-workers with all levels of ability. I would also accept a work situation where the employees were mostly people with disabilities but where the work involved a lot of engagement with the general public, such as the operation of a restaurant or a retail store. The point is that people with disabilities should have an opportunity, through their work, to overcome the segregation they used to be stuck with.

The Rehab Act specifies that supported employment is for people with "the most severe disabilities" because it envisions ongoing assistance at the job site, a level of support many people with mild disabilities may not need. That level of support is, as the next point of the definition indicates, more intensive or more extended than the usual rehabilitation service.

The majority of vocational rehabilitation is for the purpose of getting people back to work after their employment has been interrupted by illness or disease. Supported employment services, on the other hand, may require one-to-one support (job coaching) for many months to allow full employment for a person whose disability has kept her from working.

ADA—AMERICANS WITH DISABILITIES ACT

Another piece of U.S. legislation that has been of great help in supporting full employment for people with disabilities is the Americans with Disabilities Act (ADA) of 1990. Ten years after its enactment, the ADA's impact on employment for people with disabilities is still being worked out in court decisions and administrative rulings. The important thing for you to know about the ADA is that it prohibits employers from discriminating against people simply because they have a disability.

The ADA, and all the court rulings that have followed, seeks to balance two competing concerns—"reasonable accommodation" and "undue hardship."

A "reasonable accommodation" is any change in the job site that would allow a person with disabilities to do the job. Some of the more obvious accommodations are things like work tables that are the right height for wheelchairs, or automatically opening doors in bathrooms. Less obvious, but more important to people who have developmental disabilities, are things like picture job task charts or simple assembly jigs.

"Undue hardship" is what an employer claims when he thinks the accommodation will cost too much or unfairly disrupt the work area. As a job coach, you may ask for an accommodation you think is reasonable, and the employer may reply that that is an undue hardship. If these cases cannot be worked out, they can end up in court.

When we were doing Access, Inc. services, the country was in a time of unprecedented prosperity. Entry level jobs were going begging, and employers had a hard time finding and keeping reliable workers. Employers were very willing to make whatever accommodations will allow a reliable worker to do good work. As unemployment has risen in the past year, it has become harder to find those jobs. But many employers, having learned about the reliability and productivity of workers with disabilities, have stuck with them.

VOLUNTEERING

Volunteer work can have some of the same positive effects as competitive employment, while having less pressure. A person who says he doesn't want to get a job may have had bad experience with work. A volunteer job allows him to get used to getting up in the morning, being dressed appropriately, following instructions, and getting along with others. Volunteer work allows a person to meet other volunteers and to show that he has something to offer his community. The only rule is that the work must be the kind that other people volunteer for. It's exploitative and illegal for an employer to get a person to work as a "volunteer" at a job someone else would be paid for.

Lisa said she absolutely didn't want a job. But she agreed to work with her community coach three mornings a week sorting clothes at the Salvation Army homeless shelter. The woman who ran the shelter was impressed with Lisa's neatness and attention to detail, so she introduced Lisa to a friend of hers who was looking for someone to organize displays in her clothing shop. Volunteering led Lisa to a job she now loves and to the status of "valued employee."

FIVE STEPS TO EFFECTIVE JOB COACHING

Helping a person with disabilities on the job is called "job coaching." Some people think job coaching is a specialized service that requires specialized training and education (you can even get a master's degree in it). I disagree. I think a job coach needs the same attitudes and skills needed for supporting a person in any other life activity. As a job coach you are gradually nudging a person with disabilities into the mainstream of life.

There is, however, a specialized field of supported employment and rehabilitation services. If you are going to be a job coach, you might want to check out some of the additional resources listed at the back of this book. You will also need to know the steps of what is the "standard" supported employment service:

- Assessment
- Vocational Plan
- Job Development
- On-the-job Training
- Fading

ASSESSMENT

As we have seen, every type of support program starts out with an assessment. You have to know where you are in order to know where to go.

There are lots of very technical vocational assessment tools on the market. In the hands of a trained professional, these devices can gather good information about a person's physical and mental abilities, what jobs he might be capable of, and what kinds of accommodations he might need.

My issue with these assessment tools is that they often don't lead to understanding of who the potential employee is. What are his hopes for the future? How does he see himself? What support resources does he already have? What does work mean to him? Why does he want to work? What would his "perfect" job be, even if that goal is not "realistic?" These are the kinds of things you learn about a person as you get to know him, as he opens up to you and you build a relationship of trust and mutual respect. No tests or checklists can get at the things that are really important.

When we started Access, Inc. we were seen as not being "professional" job coaches. One of the ways people challenged me was to ask what kind of vocational assessment we were using. I told them we had developed an assessment device of our own. We asked the person, "Where do you think you'd like to work?" If she said, "Bojangles," we'd go with her down to Bojangles and help her put in an application.

This really happened. Ethel kept insisting she wanted to work at Bojangles. The case management professionals tried to convince her that that was not an "appropriate" job for her. She pitched tantrums, ran away from home, and refused to do any work at the workshop. Finally, we advocated enough for her that she was "allowed" to apply at Bojangles. Her application was accepted, and she started to work the following day.

After about an hour of work, she told her job coach, "I can't work here. It stinks like grease." The job coach used this realization as an opportunity to help Ethel learn how to tell the manager she quit. And then the job coach helped Ethel start her job history.

Some employment specialists believe that if we had done an adequate assessment we would have found Ethel's perfect job for her right off the bat. When I heard this criticism I would ask the critic, "Is this your first job?" Invariably it wasn't. We all go through many jobs before we find what's right for us, often by painful trial and error. There's no shortcut that will save a person with disabilities from this process that is part of real life in the real world.

VOCATIONAL PLAN

An assessment, of course, leads to a plan. A Vocational Plan will list the kinds of work the person wants and the supports she will need for success. It should be part of the larger person-centered plan. Planning for a job cannot be done in isolation from other concerns like where to live, whether to go to school and who a person's friends are.

A Vocational Plan should also address the issue of money management. Real work produces real income. Even working 20 hours a week at $5.50 an hour yields $110 a week. That's a lot of money to a person who is used to making $50 a month at the workshop. He will need a plan for budgeting his money, and he will need support for understanding the impact of his earnings on the disability benefits he receives. Fortunately, this latter is not as much a problem as it used to be. The Work Incentives Improvement Act of 1998 significantly raised the amount of money a person with disabilities could earn before losing his Medicaid benefits.

The plan should list outcomes, benchmarks by which we can measure whether or not we are doing our jobs well. If one of Hazel's goals is to work at Bojangles, then one of the plan's outcomes should be "Hazel will get a job at Bojangles." Then it should list what we should do to make that happen.

The plan will also have to be flexible. I don't know about you, but I never had a clear career plan. I took opportunities as they arose, changed my mind when I got bored, followed friends to places they liked. If we remember that the person is the driver of the plan, we will change the plan as needed, to reflect changes in what the person wants.

JOB DEVELOPMENT

"Job Development" is the term used to describe the process of developing employment opportunities for people with disabilities. Job Development is largely an educational process. A lot of times you have to educate potential employers about the advantages of hiring people with disabilities. Many employers think people with disabilities can't work or belong in sheltered work facilities.

Job Development can take the form of large, public advertising campaigns or can be the result of quiet, behind-the-scenes work. Once employers realize people with disabilities are a valuable employment resource, they will spread the word. One effective method I've seen is to have an annual awards banquet where an "Employer of the Year" is recognized for her efforts in making the accommodations necessary for people with disabilities to be able to work at competitive jobs. The employer gets good publicity and becomes an effective spokesperson for employment of people with disabilities.

Individual job development is as simple as helping the person you support look through the classified ads or driving around looking for "Now Hiring" signs. Use the same resources you would use if you were looking for a job—newspapers, libraries, the Yellow Pages, the Employment Security Commission, friends and family. If you are being truly supportive, you won't be looking to "place" the person in a job, you will be helping him find a job that meets his current needs.

JOBSITE TRAINING

Once a person finds a job, she has to learn how to do it. That's true for anyone on any job. Do you remember the first day at work on some of your previous jobs? There are papers to fill out, people to meet, procedures to learn. It can be pretty scary.

As a job coach, your role on the jobsite is the same as when you are supporting someone in any other activity. You give only as much support as is needed. You use good teaching techniques. You set up accommodations as necessary. Then you try to stay out of the way.

FADING

Your ultimate goal in job coaching, as in every other kind of support, is to eventually fade away. In fact, that's what the last of the five steps of job coaching is—fading.

Fading your support as a job coach doesn't mean the person will not need any support on the job. Fading just means that she won't need you, as a paid job coach, to be with her on the job. Does that mean that she won't need any support or assistance? Of course not. She may always need a little extra help with some things. Fading means you have done your job coaching so well that you have helped her set up natural supports at work.

You will always run into some people who are prejudiced against people with disabilities. You may be able to change their attitude by your example, or they may make the job so miserable for the person you support that he has to leave. Usually, though, you meet people just like you and me, caring people who are anxious to give a good co-worker the support he needs. Try to identify these people early and help the person you support cultivate a closer relationship with them. The day will come when the co-worker will say to you, "You know, I don't think he really needs you to come to the job anymore. I think I can give him whatever little help he needs. We're getting to be pretty good friends." That's when you'll know that your job coaching work is done and you can move on to help bring success to someone else.

AFFIRMATIVE ENTERPRISES

Just as many people's ultimate residential goal is to own their own home, many people's highest vocational objective is to own their own business. If a person is having trouble getting the community to accept her as an employee, maybe she can take the big step and be her own boss.

At Access, Inc. we helped people with disabilities partner with others to form businesses that provided communities with needed services. People started a pet grooming business, an office supplies store, and a car washing service. One woman and her coach formed a residential cleaning business. One of the high points of my career was the day those two cut the ribbon at a Chamber of Commerce grand opening ceremony. I had watched as these two women, one of whom had spent many years in public mental health facilities, discovered their strengths and developed the courage to become entrepreneurs.

Housing and employment are the biggest areas in which people with disabilities have been shoved to the edges and kept out of the mainstream. So they are the best openings to inclusion. When you help someone set up his own home or get the job that's right for him, you have overcome many of the barriers to real life in the real world.

Chapter 14

WHAT'S LOVE GOT TO DO WITH IT?

The idea of love being important to our work has not been much respected in the field of disabilities support. We're a little afraid of it. We're afraid it might lead to the cutesy falseness of "Jerry's kids," playing on shallow sympathy and seeing people with disabilities as cuddly children. And our scientific, clinical side thinks love is just entirely too mushy and soft. It will never be able to confront the hard problems and issues we face every day. Then there's the issue of "professional distance." I was taught not to get too close to the people I supported. Some of my professional colleagues at Colin Anderson Center expressed concern that by bringing Billy and Lloyd into my home I was in danger of losing my "objectivity." As if what I had to offer as a professional should be like medicine, dispensed in regular, equal doses to all.

I've wrestled with those issues, but I've finally come down on the side of love. I've decided *love is the most important aspect of our work*. It's what gives our work power and meaning and effectiveness. Love is like fertilizer—it makes living things grow and bloom.

This realization was driven home to me shortly before I started writing this book. I mentioned earlier that I like to travel around and see what other people in our field are up to. One person I had heard about but never seen was John McGee. John is the developer of what he calls "Gentle Teaching." He says it is "for those who want to uncover ways to express companionship instead of control." I had the opportunity to travel to Charlotte, NC to see an introductory workshop John was presenting. When I got there, the place was packed. I sat in the back, ready to take notes, ready to be my usual critical self. I did take notes, but I wrote because I was moved and inspired.

The high point of that day for me was a video of John working with a woman who lived in a facility in Europe. The woman was dressed in what appeared to be a hospital gown. She was crouched on the floor in the corner of an empty room. She was making low, humming noises and tearing up bits of paper or cloth. She was obviously frightened, isolated, and angry. As the film crew recorded from the doorway, John went in and sat quietly next to the woman. He smiled. He talked in a low and reassuring way. He joined her in picking up some of the torn pieces. When she yelled and tried to hit him, he backed off. When she accepted his presence, he reached out and touched her gently on the shoulder. I was spellbound. I saw that all of my clinical experience and book-learning, all the things I thought I'd figured out, boiled down to this—one human being reaching out to another. Simply for the love of it. It's as simple as that.

SEPARATION AND LOSS

People who have disabilities did not drop onto this planet from spaceships. They were born here, welcomed into our human family, loved by parents and siblings. Those who stay in that loving atmosphere grow up to live lives marked by lifelong relationships and notable successes. But, as you have learned, the history of our dealings with those among us who are seen as different and strange is to separate them from family and community—either for their own good or for ours. The woman in the John McGee film was scared and alone, a condition that happens too often to people whose way of relating to the world puts other people off. When people are separated from love, they often withdraw into themselves for protection. This withdrawal cuts them off even further from the relationships that make them skillful and healthy, and they get worse—justifying their removal.

Sometimes people who don't receive enough nourishing love lash out at those around them. They try to hurt people. They destroy things in fits of what seems like rage. They are prickly and tense and hard to approach.

Some people who are extremely sensitive to the pain of separation and loss (maybe wired that way) may injure themselves (SIB) to trick their emotional sensors into accepting the lesser, physical pain in place of the unendurable inner pain. I have seen people in institutional environments injure themselves over and over, crying and hurting and withdrawing.

I said early in this book that the three most important characteristics of the institutional attitude were "segregation, segregation, segregation." Remember that an institution is not a place. A person doesn't have to be sent away to be separated. That separation also occurs when children are put in "special" classes or sent to "special" camps. Separation happens when a person can't keep up, when the real world passes her by, leaving her alone and scared.

I have come to realize that much of the angry behavior I've seen over the years, the hitting and biting, the screaming and breaking, came from people who had no deep connections with others. And I remember the times I've seen parents or siblings or old friends come to visit people in segregated facilities. The squeals of delight from someone who usually sat quietly alone. The hugs and kisses. The joy at experiencing loving human contact.

We have hurt people by separating them from love. It's time to make amends.

LOVE AS TREATMENT

Lest my hard-nosed, scientific friends think I've gone entirely soft in the head, I have some intellectual reasons for my emphasis on love. About a year ago I read one of those books that once in a while comes along and changes your worldview. Titled *A General Theory of Love* (listed in the Resources section), this book was no New Age fantasy. It was written by a trio of psychiatrists and neurological researchers, and it reviews a lot of the recent scientific discoveries about how our brains and emotions work.

The idea that most astounded me from that book can be summed up in a single quote: "Love alters the structure of our brains." Imagine! These scientists are saying that research shows love to be a real force, a force that changes the way people think, feel and respond to life. When a child lives with abuse and rejection his brain develops in a way to cope with that kind of world. If the child lives with love, his brain grows and stretches and becomes all it can. Loving relationships actually increase the amount of connection in the brain and can help heal serious diseases.

Likewise, the lack of love causes brain changes that can be seen. Adults who go through some terrible event like war or rape, who have what we call post traumatic stress disorder (PTSD), show changes in their brains that show up on a PET scan. The brains of people who do not have love in their lives show decreased activity. People who live without love often wither and sometimes even die.

Ever since we came up with the idea that people who have mental retardation have something "wrong" with their brains, we sought a treatment that could overcome the damage. We have experimented with physical exercises, surgery, stimulus-response training, drugs, and shock therapy. None of these brought really significant positive results and some of them had terrible negative effects.

In recent years we've discovered the positive effects of community inclusion and self-determination. We've had a hard time providing scientific studies that prove these are good things; but we know they are. We can watch people bloom when they are put in control of their own lives and included in real life in the real world.

Now these scientists come along and tell us there is evidence that the most effective thing we are doing is providing love, connection and protection. It's just what John McGee says: "People want to feel loved and safe."

LOVE AND ATTACHMENT

Vague, generalized love will not do. We can't be like Charles Schulz' Lucy who once said, "I love humanity. It's people I can't stand." Love has to come in the form of strong bonds with particular people.

Psychologists sometimes call these bonds "attachment," and there is much evidence that problems with attachment are at the root of many life difficulties. I used to think the big issue was "relationships," as if these were something someone could be trained for, like "independent living" or "using public transportation." The studies on love and attachment, however, have helped me see that the kind of attachment that is healthy, that brings the benefits of love, is person specific. You can have a relationship with the person at the convenience store who sells you gas, but you won't have an attachment. Attachments are long-term, reliable relationships based on trust and affection.

If you are doing this job just to receive a paycheck, you will move on when a better job opens up. Your work won't be very effective. But if you are doing this job "for the love of it" (*and*, hopefully, a good paycheck), you can lay the groundwork for people who have been damaged by isolation. You can help them form real attachments, the kind that will last a lifetime, the kind that change people's brains.

SUPPORTIVE RELATIONSHIPS

Let's call what you can do a "supportive relationship." That's not as hot as "love of my life," but it reflects the reality that you have a paid, professional relationship with the person you support, rather than a deep, personal one. Hot or not, your supportive relationship can be extremely important. To a person who doesn't have much experience with life, supportive relationships can serve as emotional training wheels, holding her up until she learns to ride on her own.

My Dad didn't believe in training wheels. He thought they made kids dependent on them and kept them from learning to ride. So every time I wanted to try to ride my new Schwinn, I had to have an adult hold me up. One afternoon, my Mom was doing the support, keeping a gentle, protective hand on the back of my bicycle seat. I pedaled furiously, trying to get the hang of it. As we passed Mrs. Lake's house, Mom paused to wave at our neighbor. For a brief moment, she let go of the seat of my bike, and I, not knowing the steadying hand was gone, rode off without her. It was an exhilarating moment for both of us.

When your patient support leads to a person developing a new skill, especially one that leads to healthy, loving relationships, you have every reason to burst with pride. While you are supporting her, she learns trust, interdependence, how to ask for help, how to take care of someone else. Once she knows these things by heart, she can ride on her own.

DEVELOPING YOUR CAPACITY TO LOVE

There are several skills you have to have in order to provide this loving support. Maybe I should call them "personal characteristics" rather than skills, because I don't know if you can learn them. They may be something you bring to the job—and they should be characteristics people who make hiring decisions are looking for. If you have these things in your heart, though, your work may help you bring them out. These characteristics include:

- Attention
- Understanding
- Reliability
- Friends

ATTENTION

Modern lives are very busy. There are so many things that demand our attention—sometimes we feel driven to distraction. And we are surrounded by people whose attention is also pulled in a million different directions. We hear that thousands of kids are medicated in school for "attention deficit disorder.". Attention may be one of the biggest issues of our century.

Doesn't it mean the world to you when another person is willing to close out all of the other demanding noise and focus his attention solely on you? It makes you feel important and worthwhile and alive. We are attracted to people who are capable of offering this kind of attention. They become our close friends, our lovers.

Now imagine how important attention is to someone whose own brain is driving her to distraction or someone who has spent his days in "programs," where the attention is divided among dozens of other demanding people. We have already discussed how a lot of the challenging behavior we see is because people are demanding the attention they need. If you are the kind of person who can give that attention, you will not be beaten by the frenzy of their demands.

No matter where you work, whether in residential facilities or vocational supports or in a classroom, find time every day to give your undivided attention to each person you work with. Look into each person's eyes. Touch a hand or a shoulder. Ask how he is. See and appreciate the beauty in each one.

As you pay close attention, you will find new things to appreciate about each person you meet. And you will find new things in yourself, as well.

UNDERSTANDING

When I was in Basic Aide Training, I wanted to know "Who are these 'retarded kids'?" As if "they" were some simple quantity to be known, like the specs of a fast car.

I found that people with developmental disabilities are sometimes hard to know and understand. Particularly when someone doesn't use words for communication or when their words are hard to follow, you will have to pay very close attention. But then you will have to try to understand what it is like to be that person. How does the world seem to the man who is always lying down and looking up? How does the young woman with severe cerebral palsy feel when an IQ test suddenly discovers she's smart? What is in the heart of the man whose physical appearance is such that small children, upon seeing him, run and hide behind their mothers?

"Empathy" is the word used for the ability to truly and deeply understand how another person feels. If you can develop your ability to be empathetic, all your relationships will benefit—and people who have been misunderstood or ignored will be drawn to you for life.

RELIABILITY

One of the most important learning tasks for the person who has been regularly abandoned and betrayed, either early on by family members or later by the system, is trust. Many, many people with disabilities have been lied to, fooled and betrayed. I have met people who don't trust anyone, who feel alone against the world.

You will hear trust problems referred to as "adjustment disorders" or "attachment disorders." Those are fine psychological terms, but they don't lead to a cure. The only way a person can learn to trust is by being in the company of someone who is trustworthy and reliable. You can be that person. You can be the supportive relationship that leads a person back to a sense of trust. You're never going to get people to trust "the system," no matter how many institutional changes occur. But if they trust you, they may become open to new opportunities.

FRIENDS

I know, friends aren't really a personal characteristic. But the fact that you have a wide circle of friends tells me something about you. It tells me that you understand interdependence, even if you never heard that word before you read this book. The fact that you have a personal network tells me you know how to set one up. You know how to be a friend—to send cards when someone is sick, to pick out a great birthday gift, to take photos of special occasions. You know when to offer advice and when to shut up and listen. You have the kind of "social intelligence" that draws people to you.

Once I was interviewing a woman for a position as a community coach. She said, apologetically, that she had never done this kind of work before. Then she added, "My husband says I just love people too much. Our house is always full, and I never turn anyone away." I knew right then that she was going to be very successful as a coach.

Now that you're fired up about how great you are, let me give you a little warning. If you are a paid support provider, you cannot become the best friend of the person you support. You can show him how to *be* a friend and how to *have* a friend. You can make sure he gets to the places where he can meet people who might become his friend. But you are the training wheels only. Be proud when he has his own friends, lots of them, people he can count on for the rest of his life.

WHAT'S LOVE GOT TO DO WITH IT?

I said at the beginning of this chapter that you don't hear much about love in this business. Well, that's not entirely true. Things are changing. I have heard speakers at several recent conferences refer to the importance of love.

Love is coming into the mainstream of the disability support field. I think it will be the power behind the next wave that takes us into the future.

And you are at the right place to ride that wave. You know about the past and will not be doomed to repeat its mistakes. You know about how we usually do things today and are primed for success, wherever you work. But most importantly, you have your eyes on the future. Do good work. Let me know how it comes out.

APPENDIX I

GLOSSARY OF TERMS

abnormal—not the usual or average (see **normal** and **atypical**)

accommodation—an adjustment that makes an environment more suitable, convenient or accessible. "Reasonable accommodations" are required by the ADA to make places of employment and other public facilities accessible to people with disabilities.

accessible—able to be reached or used, open, available

ADA—Americans with Disabilities Act (1991)

ADL—activities of daily living

adaptive skills—skills needed to adapt (adjust) to everyday life; sometimes measured through the use of "adaptive behavior scales"

adjudicated incompetent—determined by a court of law to be incapable of making certain kinds of personal decisions. A guardian will be appointed to assist with the areas of incompetence.

advocacy—speaking out or working on behalf of someone whose rights have been threatened or violated

affective—relating to **moods** and emotions

aggression—in behavioral terms, any action that hurts or threatens to hurt another person. Usually includes hitting, kicking, biting, spitting at, throwing objects at or verbally threatening.

akathisia—restlessness sometimes experienced as an effect of medication

ambulation, ambulatory—walking or moving about, able to walk

amnesia—loss of memory

Antecedent—what comes before a **behavior** and causes it to happen

antecedent reinforcer—giving a reward before the behavior is completed—not a good way to motivate behavior

anticholinergic (ant-ee-cole-in-URGE-ic)—affecting the functioning of acetylcholine (a **neurotransmitter**) in the body. Anticholinergic side effects to certain drugs include such **symptom**s as dry mouth, constipation and dizziness.

anticonvulsant—having the effect of controlling **seizures** (convulsions)

anxiety disorder—mental health disorder marked by feelings of fear, dread, worry, **compulsive** behavior and flashbacks of stressful events

aphasia (uh-FAY-zhuh)– an **impairment** of the ability to use or comprehend words, usually acquired as a result of a stroke or other brain injury

assess—to evaluate

Asperger's Disorder—marked by **impairments** in social interactions and the presence of restricted interests and activities, with no clinically significant general delay in language, and testing in the range of average to above average intelligence

atypical—not what is usually expected

auditory—having to do with the ears or hearing

Autism—a brain disorder that impairs the ability to communicate, socialize, and maintain ordinary relationships with others. People with autism demonstrate a range of verbal and intellectual capacities, from low to high. They also demonstrate a broad range of **symptom**s. Children with autism may, for instance, resist even minor changes in their routines. They may also appear detached or withdrawn in social situations, unable to engage in ordinary conversation. In severe cases of autism, children may make repetitive body movements such as rocking; they may also engage in aggressive and self-injurious behavior such as biting their own hands.

barbiturate—a class of addictive drugs used as sedatives (to calm anxiety or produce sleep), reduce pain, or control seizures (anticonvulsant). Includes Phenobarbital and Seconal.

baseline—the condition that exists before an experimental **intervention** is started. This gives a starting point from which to measure whether desired changes are occurring. Baseline **data** measures the rate at which a behavior occurs before medication or behavioral programming are started.

behavior—what a person (or animal) does, activity. Behavior can be observed, unlike feelings, **motivations** and thoughts.

Behaviorism—a school of psychology that takes observable behavior and its causes as the only concern of its research and the only basis of its theory without reference to "internal" mental states. Founders include Americans John B. Watson and B.F. Skinner.

Benzodiazepines—a class of medications, including Valium (diazepam), Librium (chlordiazepoxide), and Xanax (alprazolam), used to treat **anxiety disorders**. Highly addictive.

beta-blocker—a class of medications, including Inderal (propranolol) and Tenormin (atenolol), typically used to treat high blood pressure, irregular heartbeat and migraine headaches, but also effective for some **anxiety disorders** and unexplained outbursts of agitation or **aggression**

Bipolar disorder—an **affective** (mood) disorder having both **manic** (agitated, aroused) and **depressive** ("down," "blue") episodes, often marked by **mood** swings that may run in cycles

Borderline Personality Disorder—a lifelong style of relating to life (personality) that is marked by instability of interpersonal relationships, self-image and mood. Additional characteristics include:

- fear of abandonment
- intense swings from love to hate toward the same person
- self-damaging behavior (sex, substance abuse, reckless driving, binge eating)
- suicidal behavior and threats
- self-mutilation (cutting, burning)
- chronic feeling of emptiness and dissatisfaction with life

bowel movement—often referred to as "BM"; less professionally referred to as "poop." The medical term is "**defecate**."

categorical funding—funding that is based on a type of disability or type of service rather than the needs of a particular person (as opposed to "**participant driven**" funding)

central nervous system (CNS)—made up of the brain and spinal cord

Cerebral palsy—a group of motor disorders caused by damage to the motor areas of the brain, can cause difficulties with movement and speech

chromosomes—the bodies in cells that contain genes and determine what the cell will do. Most humans have 46 chromosomes, 23 from each parent. Occasionally, an extra chromosome (a **trisomy**) will cause abnormal development (see **genetic**).

chronic—lasting over a long period of time, or happening regularly over a period of time

chronological age—how many years the person has been on the planet

clinician—a person specializing in a particular medical field such as psychiatry, psychology, nursing, physical therapy. Usually required to complete a course of study, meet licensing requirements and adhere to ethical and best practice guidelines

cognitive—having to do with thinking processes like reasoning and logic

compulsion—behavior a person feels driven to accomplish, often without knowing why

condition—in research design, the environment the subject is in. For example, setting up the lever that delivers a reward to the pigeon each time it pecks is a condition of the experiment.

condition change—when a researcher changes the conditions of the experiment or the subject (see **variable**). This is often done to see what happens under the new conditions. For example, making it so pecking no longer brings the reward of a pellet is a "change of condition."

confidential—personal and private

Consequence—what follows (comes after) a **Behavior** and is caused by that **Behavior**

cue—an event in the environment that serves as an **Antecedent** to a particular Behavior (see **prompt**)

custodial—having to do with taking care of and being responsible for

data—pieces of information

data-based—based on recorded information about what really took place

data collection—gathering and recording accurate information, usually from observation

defecate—the correct medical term for a **bowel movement**. The resulting material is correctly called feces (fee-sees).

degenerative—getting worse over time

deinstitutionalization—the process of moving people with developmental disabilities and mental illness from large, centralized state facilities into smaller, community-based facilities

delirium—reduced clarity of awareness of what is going on in the person's life, usually of short **duration** and caused by a medical condition or substance abuse

delusion—a false, **persistent** belief that runs contrary to the experience of others; e.g., that someone is reading one's thoughts

dementia—impairment of **cognition** (thinking, understanding) that results from a medical condition or substance abuse; usually long term, often **degenerative**; is a primary **symptom** of Alzheimer's, Parkinson's, Huntington's, HIV and stroke

depression—affective (**mood**) disorder marked by a depressed ("down") mood and lack of interest in previously enjoyable activities. Additional **symptom**s may include a decline in personal hygiene, sleep disturbance, eating disturbance, irritability, feelings of worthlessness, difficulty concentrating, thoughts of suicide.

developmental disability—an **impairment** in **functioning** that results during the **developmental period**, **e.g.**, mental retardation, blindness, deafness, **cerebral palsy**

developmental milestones—things most infants and children can do at particular ages. Children who don't reach these milestones at the appropriate time may be seen as "developmentally delayed."

developmental period—the period in which a person is developing, usually from conception to age 18

deviant, deviation—different from the **normal** or usual, something that is different

diagnosis—determination, by a clinician, of which disease entity is indicated by the presenting **symptom**s

disability—an **organic malfunction** that causes physical or mental performance to be other than usually expected

discipline—a course of study, usually leading to an advanced degree or license to practice, e.g. nursing, psychology, social work

dopamine—a **neurotransmitter** involved in **mood** and the control of complex movements. The loss of dopamine activity in some portions of the brain leads to the muscular rigidity of Parkinson's disease. Many medications used to treat behavioral disorders work by modifying the action of dopamine in the brain.

Down syndrome—the most commonly occurring **genetic** condition. One in every 800 to 1,000 live births is a child with Down **syndrome**, representing approximately 5,000 births per year in the United States alone. Most people with Down syndrome have IQs in the mild to moderate range of mental retardation. The most common form of Down syndrome is called **Trisomy** 21, because it involves an extra copy of the 21st **chromosome**. People with Down syndrome have recognizable facial characteristics that make the syndrome easy to identify in infancy. There are some long-term health problems associated with Down syndrome that can cause a shortened life expectancy.

dual-diagnosis—**developmental disability** and mental illness in the same person (in substance abuse treatment, this refers to substance abuse and mental illness)

due process— the right to be heard in court, to bring lawsuits, to have the representation of an attorney, to face our accuser and to bring witnesses on our behalf

duration—how long something lasts

dysfunction—from *dys*, meaning *hard, bad, or difficult*. **Functioning** of an organ or system in a way that is less than expected

dystonia—a **neurological** disorder marked by involuntary muscle contractions and spasms which result in abnormal postures and movements. Often accompanied by a twisting or jerking motion. It can be caused by some medications or can be due to unknown **organic** causes.

Early intervention services—services provided to infants, toddlers, young children, and their families to—
- (A) enhance the development of infants, toddlers, and young children with disabilities and to minimize their potential for **developmental** delay; and
- (B) enhance the capacity of families to meet the special needs of their infants, toddlers, and young children.

Educable—in special education, children who test in the **Mild** range of mental retardation

e.g.—"for example"

empirical—based on observation and testing, **data**-based

emotion—feeling, affect, reaction

environment—existing conditions, situation, place, surroundings

exploitation—taking unfair advantage of someone because of his or her condition or status

extinction—when a behavior stops occurring

extrapyramidal symptoms—may occur even after a few doses of a medication; these include:
- acute **dystonia** (spasms, drooling, difficulty breathing)
- Parkinsonian Syndrome (tremor, rigidity, drooling, shuffling gait)
- **akathisia** (restlessness, agitation).

fading—reducing the amount of support you give as a person is able to function more independently (see **graduated guidance**)

feces (fee-sees)—the results of a **bowel movement**

Fetal Alcohol Syndrome (FAS)—physical and neurological damage done to a developing baby in the womb when the mother drinks high levels of alcohol

fine motor—nervous system controlling small muscles such as fingers and tongue

frequency—how often something occurs

function—how something works or operates. The usual use of something is said to be its "function".

gait—manner of walking

generalization—applying skills learned in one **environment** to a new and different environment

generic name—the descriptive name of a drug, regardless of the manufacturer (as opposed to "brand name" used by the company that developed the drug and holds a patent or license). When listed together, the brand name of a drug starts with a capital letter and the generic name starts with a small letter, e.g. thioridazine (Mellaril).

genetics—the study of how information that controls the development of an organism is passed down from its parents

gestural prompt—showing a person what to do by **modeling** or pointing

graduated guidance—using only as much assistance as necessary and **fading** as the person becomes able to complete a task more independently

gross motor—nervous system controlling large muscles such as legs and arms

hallucinations—visual, seeing things that are not there; **auditory**, hearing things that are not there

handicap—the things a person has difficulty doing because of a **disability**

hemiplegia—a paralysis on one side of the body, therefore "right hemiplegia" and "left hemiplegia"

hypothesis—an educated guess that needs to be tested

ICF-MR—Intermediate Care Facility-Mental Retardation—a designation of a level of care in the Medicaid system

IDEA—Individuals with Disabilities Education Act of 1997

Idiot—outdated term for a person with an IQ of less than 25 (below **Imbecile** and **Moron**)

IEP—Individualized Education Plan, required for all special education students

IFSP—Individual Family Support Plan, required for early childhood intervention programs receiving Federal funds

Imbecile—outdated term for a person with an IQ from 25 to 50 (higher than **Idiot** and lower than **Moron**)

impairment—damage that weakens or diminishes **function**

incidental learning (also called **informal learning**)—the theory that people can learn without being formally trained. The learning occurs through participating in activities.

inclusion—a situation in which no one is segregated because of a condition he or she is not responsible for, whether the segregation is due to ignorance and fear, or to a feeling of "special" entitlement

informed consent—agreement to something based on a full understanding of the consequences of that choice. "Informed" means having and understanding the information necessary.

intensity—how strong or powerful something is

interdependence—the fact that we all rely on a network of family and friends, that none of us is completely independent

interdisciplinary team—in the Medicaid system, a team of professionals from various **disciplines** that is responsible for "active treatment" (the interdisciplinary team is headed by a "**Q**")

intervention—literally "coming between," usually referring to a program or treatment that comes between the person and some bad consequence or behavior, interruption, stepping in

LEA (Local Education Agency)—usually a local school board or district, the agency held responsible for special education services under **IDEA**

limit testing—seeing how much you can get away with, testing to see where the limits are. Occurs more frequently in situations where the limits are known to be flexible.

LRE (Least Restrictive Environment)—the place or situation where a person with disabilities can receive support services with the least loss of freedom

mainstreaming—education of children with disabilities in the same classes and schools as typical children

maladaptive—not helping a person get along in a particular **environment**, usually referring to behaviors that don't lead to desired consequences

malfunction—something wrong in the way a system operates (see **function**)

manic—agitated, aroused. A person having a "manic episode" may also exhibit:
- inflated self-esteem (grandiosity)
- decreased need for sleep
- pressured speech
- distractibility

Mental age—a measure used in psychological testing that expresses an individual's mental ability in terms of the number of years it takes an average child to reach the same level (see **chronological age**)

MI—mental illness

Mild mental retardation—marked by IQ test scores of 51-69

mobility—ability to move; sometimes used interchangeably with **ambulation**, the ability to walk

modeling—doing an activity correctly so that a person watching can learn how to do it by observation

Moderate mental retardation—marked by IQ test scores of 36-51

mood—feeling, state of mind

mood altering—changing a person's state of mind. Often used to refer to medications that deal with **mood disorders** like **depression** and **anxiety**

mood disorder—disturbances of mood that are serious enough or of long enough **duration** to require clinical **intervention**. Includes depressive disorders (marked by a "down" or "blue" mood) and bipolar disorders (which have **manic** times, in addition to depressed periods).

Moron—outdated term referring to people with an IQ of 50-75

motivation—what gets a person moving

MR—mental retardation

mutation—an unexpected change in the **genetic** information that controls how an organism will develop and **function**

natural supports—family, friends, neighbors and co-workers who can offer someone the supports and assistance he/she needs, so he/she doesn't have to rely on the disability system

neuroleptic—another term for **"antipsychotic,"** used to refer to medications that treat **psychotic** disorders

neurological—having to do with nerves or the nervous system

neurotransmitter—chemical in the brain and **central nervous system** that is responsible for communicating with and sometimes controlling other systems. Some examples are **dopamine, serotonin** and acetylcholine.

non-compliance—When a person refuses to do what he is told to do by authorized staff he may be said to be "non-compliant." Sometimes these people are put on training programs to make them more "compliant" (obedient). "Non-compliance" is not a term you would use with your family or friends. If this term is in your vocabulary you can replace it with "doesn't like to do what he's told." Just like your husband.

normal—what is usually expected, average, standard (see **deviant**)

Obsessive-compulsive disorder (OCD)—**anxiety disorder** marked by **obsessions** (**persistent** thoughts, ideas or images that are experienced as intrusive and cause anxiety and distress) and **compulsions** (repetitive behaviors or mental acts, such as hand-washing, checking, counting, the goal of which is to reduce anxiety or stress)

Obsessions—**persistent** thoughts, ideas or images that are experienced as intrusive and cause **anxiety** and distress

operant conditioning—teaching by coupling a reward with the correct performance of a task or response to a **cue**

organic—having to do with an organism, living, physiological. When talking about the cause of a **dysfunction**, "organic" means coming from inside the person, as opposed to "**environmental**," being caused by outside factors

outcome—a result or **consequence**. Something that happens in a person's life that makes a difference to him/her.

panic attack—an episode of fear or discomfort, peaking quickly (within 10 minutes) and including such **symptom**s as heart palpitations, sweating, trembling and shortness of breath

pseudoparkinsonism—a condition (usually caused by a drug) that looks like Parkinson's disease, marked by tremor and weakness of resting muscles and by a shuffling **gait**

paralysis—loss of the ability to move a part of the body

paraplegia—paralysis of the lower half of the body

participant driven supports—another term for **self-determination**. A system in which the person receiving support services (the "participant") is in the driver's seat.

pathology—the **functional** and structural changes caused by a disease

perception—awareness that comes through the senses and is interpreted by the brain

persistent—continuing to exist without change, constant

pervasive—having effects throughout all areas of a person's life

Phenothiazine—a group of drugs used to treat serious mental and emotional disorders, including **schizophrenia** and other **psychotic** disorders. Includes Mellaril (thioridazine), Prolixin (fluphenazine), and Thorazine (chlorpromazine). Some are used also to control agitation, severe nausea and vomiting, severe hiccups, and moderate to severe pain in some hospitalized patients. Phenothiazines can cause serious long-term and short-term side effects, including **extrapyramidal** symptoms, **pseudoparkinsonism**, and **tardive dyskinesia**.

Phenobarbital—a **barbiturate** drug used as a **sedative** and **anticonvulsant**, highly addictive

phobias—**persistent**, irrational, and excessive fear of some particular thing or situation (agoraphobia—fear of going out in public; claustrophobia—fear of enclosed places; acrophobia—fear of heights; arachnophobia—fear of spiders)

physical prompt—moving a person's body to get him started on a task or activity. Hand over hand assistance.

physiological—having to do with the **functions** and processes of an organism

pica—from the Latin word for magpie; eating things that are not food, such as paper, clothing, chalk

PKU—phenylketonuria, an inborn metabolic disorder that makes a newborn baby unable to digest phenylalanine (a commonly found protein). If untreated a build-up of toxins can cause brain damage and disability.

Post-traumatic stress disorder (PTSD)—an **anxiety disorder** resulting from an extreme traumatic event (such as war or sexual abuse). **Symptom**s may include reliving the stressful event ("flashbacks"), avoidance of situations that remind the person of the stressful event, and chronic anxiety, fear or agitation.

process—what a support agency *does*—reviews, procedures, documentation, etc. (as opposed to **outcomes**, which are what results from implementing the processes)

profound mental retardation—marked by IQ scores below 20

prompt—an **Antecedent** that indicates it is time to perform some action

prompting sequence—Ask (**verbal** prompt), Show (**gestural** prompt), Assist (physical prompt); used to support maximum independence

prosthetic—the replacement of a non-functioning body part with an artificial substitute

psychodynamic—having to do with the inner workings of the mind; the school of psychology started by Freud. Sometimes criticized by **behavioral psychology** as being unscientific hocus pocus.

psychosis—a type of mental disorder marked by **delusions**, **hallucinations**, disorganized speech and/or disorganized behavior; included are **schizophrenia** and **schizoaffective** disorder

psychotic—having to do with **psychosis**

psychotropic—any substance that alters thought, feeling, or behavior

punisher—something a person (or animal) doesn't like and will work to avoid. According to behavioral psychology, when a punisher follows a behavior, the **frequency** of the behavior will decrease.

Q—short term for the head of a Medicaid treatment team (QMRP, QDDP, QMHP, QSAP). The Q stands for "Qualified" (having a four-year college degree and some years experience in the relevant field). The P stands for "Professional." And the letters in between stand for the area of specialty—Mental Retardation, Developmental Disability, Mental Health, Substance Abuse.

quadriplegia—from the Latin "quad" which refers to "four"—paralysis in all four limbs (arms and legs)

redirection—getting a person to stop engaging in one sort of behavior by getting him/her involved in doing something else

reinforcer—something a person (or animal) likes and will work for; if it follows a behavior, the behavior is more likely to occur again

reinforcer preference—the things a particular person likes and will work for

Rett's Disorder—a genetic disorder which occurs almost exclusively in girls (male fetuses with the disorder seldom survive). Following a period of normal development the child begins to lose previously acquired skills, especially the use of the hands. Marked by repetitive hand movements ("hand wringing"), often beginning at the age of 1-4 years.

Rh incompatibility—develops when there is a difference in Rh blood type of the pregnant mother (Rh negative) and that of the fetus (Rh positive). May cause disorders ranging from destruction of red blood cells to hearing loss, seizures and decreased mental ability. Almost completely preventable with the use of RhoGAM test

risk/benefits analysis—weighing whether the benefits of a particular course of action outweigh the risks involved

rumination—bringing partially digested food up into the mouth and chewing it again; a form of self-stimulation

schizoaffective disorder—**psychotic** disorder marked by **delusions** and **hallucinations and** a **mood** disorder (**depression, mania,** etc.)

schizophrenia—**psychotic** disorder marked by **delusions, hallucinations** and disorganized thinking and behavior; **duration** is generally longer than 6 months

scoliosis—curvature of the spine

seclusion—when a person is put in a room by himself, usually to calm him or to protect others from harm

Appendix 1 - Glossary of Terms

sedative—causing calm and relaxation, sometimes leading to sleep

seizures—storms of electrical activity in the brain. Can cause symptoms ranging from brief staring spells to life threatening episodes that cause falls and breathing difficulties.

self-contained classroom—a classroom made up entirely of special education children. As opposed to **mainstreaming**.

self stim—short for "self stimulation." Purposeless, repetitive activities engaged in by people who live in non-stimulating (institutional) environments. Some examples are rocking, finger gazing, making repetitive sounds.

serotonin—a **neurotransmitter** that plays a role in elevating **mood**, regulating sleep and body temperature, and normalizing eating behavior, all of which helps to keep a person emotionally balanced.

Serotonin Reuptake Inhibitor (SSRI)—a class of medications (including Prozac, Zoloft, and Paxil) that raises levels of **serotonin** in the nervous system. Used to treat **depression**, **obsessive-compulsive disorder**, PMS, some eating disorders and other **mood disorders**.

Severe mental retardation—marked by IQ test scores of 20-35

SIB—self-injurious behavior

spatial—having to do with things in space, as location, shape or relationship

state disorder—a condition that comes and goes; as opposed to a **trait disorder** which stays the same throughout one's life. State disorders are indicated on Axis I in the multi-axial diagnosis system.

stereotype—from the Greek "stereo," which means "hard or fixed," thus, a rigid or fixed way of thinking about an issue or group of people

stereotypical behavior—purposeless, repetitive actions (rocking, light gazing, finger flying, etc.). Sometimes called "**self stim**."

stimulus—a change or event that excites a reaction or response

symptom—an indication or sign that something is wrong. Fever and chills are "symptoms" of the flu. (see **syndrome** and **diagnosis**)

syndrome—a number of **symptom**s occurring together and characterizing a particular disease

tardive dyskinesia—a late onset movement disorder, caused by long-term use of some **psychotropic** medications, presenting **symptom**s of facial grimacing, random chewing movement, and uncontrolled movement in head, arms and legs. This condition cannot be cured or reversed.

target behavior—the challenging behavior that is supposed to be reduced by a programmatic **intervention**

task analysis—breaking a complicated activity (washing hands, for example) into smaller steps that can be learned one step at a time

TBI—traumatic brain injury

Trainable—in Special Education a student in the Moderate range of mental retardation

trait disorder—a long-term disorder in the way a person relates to the world. Includes mental retardation and personality disorders, and is indicated on Axis II of the multi-axial diagnostic system.

transitional services—helping a young person move from school into the adult world of work and home

trisomy—a gene that has three ("tri") **chromosomes** instead of the usual two. A common cause of birth disorders.

Universal Language—the language we use with our family and friends and that they use with us

variable—in research, a **condition** that is changed to find out what impact the change has on the research subject

verbal prompt—asking someone to do something

visual—having to do with the eyes or seeing

APPENDIX II: RESOURCES

(WHERE TO GO FOR MORE INFORMATION)

Internet: Many of the resources listed below are websites on the Internet. These are the best places to go for the latest information, answers to questions, and contacts with other people in the field. If you don't have a computer, most libraries do. I've chosen the sites I've found most helpful or interesting.

A good place to start on the Internet is the Quality Mall (www.qualitymall.org) maintained by the Research and Training Center on Community Living of the University of Minnesota. Quoting from the directory page of that site: *Welcome to Quality Mall, a place where you can find lots of free information about person-centered supports for people with developmental disabilities. Each of the Mall stores has departments you can look through to learn about positive practices that help people with developmental disabilities live, work and participate in our communities and improve the quality of their supports.*

Books: You can find books that are about general topics or ones that are about very specific, specialized areas. Some are written only for professional clinicians, but many are written for laypeople, family and friends of people with disabilities. I have found those books listed below to be particularly helpful and accessible, but you can find others in your public library, local bookseller, or from the Internet.

Organizations: The websites of most organizations have links to other websites that have useful information about the topic the organization addresses. You can also get a feel for the organization and whether membership would be helpful to you. Some will even let you join online. Membership in these organizations usually gets you a newsletter or e-mail alert that tells about their conferences and meetings.

Conferences: Conferences and conventions, whether international, national, or regional are great places to hear speakers on all kinds of topics. You can also meet other people who are engaged in the same kind of work as you. If you get a chance to go to a big conference, jump at it.

MENTAL RETARDATION AND DEVELOPMENTAL DISABILITIES

Yahoo's Disability and the Disabled web page: *http://dailynews.yahoo.com/full_coverage/world/disabilities_and_the_disabled/* Lots of links to other interesting sites.

National Down Syndrome Society *(www.ndss.org)* a comprehensive, on-line information source about Down syndrome.

Down Syndrome Health Issues *(www.ds-health.com)* Developed by Len Leshin, M.D., F.A.A.P., the father of Avi, 6 years old, and Nathan, 8 years old. Avi's Down Syndrome inspired Dr. Leshin to write these essays about children with Down Syndrome for other parents.

Epilepsy foundation *(www.efa.org)*: "to work for children and adults affected by seizures through research, education, advocacy and service".

United Cerebral Palsy *(www.ucpa.org)*

FASLink *(www.acbr.com/fas)* this site gives complete information about Fetal Alcohol Syndrome.

PUBLISHERS

Diverse City Press *(www.diverse-city.com)* "Diverse City Press is a small publishing company which aims to provide educational materials for people with disabilities and their care providers. The company is informed by the disability rights movement, and is closely linked with organizations and individuals fighting for the rights of all people with disabilities to take control of their own lives and control their own fate".

Attainment Company (www.attainmentcompany.com) produces training materials for people with disabilities. Videos and training materials in the areas of autism, life skills, work skills, disability awareness, and parent and professional resources.

Inclusion Press *(www.inclusion.com)* "a small independent press striving to produce readable, accessible, user-friendly books and resources about full inclusion in school, work, and community".

MIND, BRAIN, AND INTELLIGENCE

BrainConnection.com *(www.brainconnection.com)* is dedicated to providing accessible, high-quality information about how the brain works and how people learn. With links to NPR's "The Infinite Mind," "Ask Dr. Expert," and "Neuro News".

The Infinite Mind from NPR is "a weekly public radio show focusing on the art and science of the human mind and spirit, behavior, and mental health." At their website, *www.theinfinitemind.com*, you can get tapes, transcripts, and program schedules.

An Anthropologist on Mars, Alfred A. Knopf, 1995; Awakenings, Harper Perennial, 1990 and The Man who Mistook his Wife for a Hat, Summit Books, 1985—These fascinating books by the neurologist Oliver Sacks are interesting explorations of the way disease or accident can affect behavior and understanding, which gives insights into how the mind works.

The Mismeasure of Man, Stephen Jay Gould. A good history of some of the wacky notions people have had about measuring intelligence.

The Bell Curve, Richard J. Herrnstein and Charles Murray. This 1995 study caused a huge amount of controversy with its exploration of intelligence, race, and social class.

Intelligence Reframed, Martin Gardner. An exploration of the theory of multiple intelligences, by the MIT professor who first came up with the idea.

Emotional Intelligence, Daniel Groleman. Building on Gardner's multiple intelligences, Groleman explores one particular way of being "smart"—emotional intelligence.

A General Theory of Love, T. Lewis, F. Amini, and R. Lannon, Random House, 2000 Discussed in Chapter 14, "What's Love Got To Do With It?"

MENTAL ILLNESS AND ITS TREATMENTS

Mental Health Aspects of Developmental Disabilities, *(www.mhaspectsofdd.com)*—the website for ordering an interesting newsletter, published by some of the leading experts in the field

Mental Health Net *(www.cmhcsys.com)*—news, reviews and resources

Schizophrenia: *Surviving Schizophrenia—A manual for Families, Consumers and Providers*, E. Fuller Torry, MD, Harper Perennial, 1995.

Bi-polar Disorder: *An Unquiet Mind*, Kay Redfield Jamison, Vintage Paperback, 1995.

Borderline Personality Disorder: *I Hate You; Don't Leave Me*, Jerold J. Kreisman, MD, Avon Books, 1989.

Internet Mental Health *(www.mentalhealth.com)* is a free encyclopedia of mental health information. Designed by a Canadian psychiatrist, Dr. Phillip Long. Information on "the 54 most common mental disorders," medication and treatment, and how diagnostic categories are different in different countries.

Mental Health: A Report of the Surgeon General *(www.surgeongeneral.gov/library/mentalhealth/)* I know that's a long address, but this US government report contains valuable information on the public health approach to mental health, including issues of diagnosis and treatment, social stigma, and mental health care financing.

Screening For Mental Health, Inc. *(www.nmisp.org)* This non-profit organization sponsors awareness days (e.g. National Depression Screening Day) about mental health issues, including depression, alcoholism, suicide, anxiety disorders, and eating disorder. There are links to information about each disorder.

National Institute of Neurological Disorders and Stroke (NINDS) *(www.ninds.nih.gov)* This site is aimed at clinical professionals, but you may find up-to-date research information about specific brain and nervous system function disorders.

National Institute of Mental Health *(www.nimh.nih.gov)* This US Government agency sponsors research into the causes and treatments of mental disorders.

The **Public Information** page of the website of the **American Psychiatric Association (APA)** *(www.psych.org/public_info/index.html)* has valuable information on various mental illnesses and the most current treatments.

SUPPORTED EMPLOYMENT

APSE—Association for Persons in Supported Employment *(www.apse.org)*

The National Supported Employment Consortium, *(www.vcu.edu/rrtcweb/sec/)* sponsored by Paul Wehman and Grant Revell at Virginia Commonwealth University.

The Affirmative Business Alliance of North America (ABANA) *(http://home.flash.net/~abana)* is an association for businesses that provide career opportunities for people with disadvantages and/or disabilities AND people from the mainstream.

Marriott Foundation *(www.marriottfoundation.org)* "Bridges ... from school to work.®" Helping special education graduates find work in the hospitality industry.

Keys to the Workplace, Michael J. Callahan and J. Bradley Garner, Paul H. Brookes Publishing, 1997.

EveryOne Can Work (videotape), Attainment Company. This is my favorite training tape. It shows a variety of people working at various jobs. Also good for potential employers.

PSYCHOTROPIC MEDICATIONS

WebMd *(www.webmd.com)* has links for everything medical, including medications, their uses, and their side effects.

The Pill Book, Bantam (this has information on all kinds of medications, not just those used in treating mental illness)

The Essential Guide to Psychiatric Drugs, Jack M. Gorman, MD, St. Martin's Paperbacks, updated 1997.

Listening to Prozac, Peter D. Kramer, MD, Viking, 1993 (not just about Prozac, this book explores the biology of personality and the issues of psychotropic medication).

Talking Back to Prozac, Peter D. Breggin, MD, St. Martin's, 1994 (a response to Kramer's book, and the beginning of an ongoing debate).

SEXUALITY

Couples with Intellectual Disabilities Talk about Living and Loving, Karin Melberg Schwier, Woodbine House, 5615 Fishers Lane, Rockville, MD 20852 (gives voice to people talking about the role of sexuality in their lives).

YAI's "Relationship Series" consists of three videotapes that explore "The Difference Between Strangers, Acquaintances and Friends," "Becoming Acquaintances or Friends," and "Becoming Friends." More information available from YAI at 460 West 34th Street, New York, NY 10001 or call 212-563-7474 ext. 193.

David Hingsburger writes and speaks plainly (and outrageously) about sexual matters. Go see him at a conference or check out his books at Diverse City Press *(www.diverse-city.com)*.

Unspoken Desire, video produced by the Australian Film Board. This one is hard to find. I saw it on the Link channel on satellite TV (www.worldlinktv.org). It is interviews with people with disabilities about how they view their sexuality and how other people perceive them. If you ever get a chance to see it, do so.

SIECUS Bibliography. The Sex Information Education Council of the US has a very complete annotated bibliography of books about sexuality and disability at *www.siecus.org/pubs/biblio.*

EARLY CHILDHOOD/SPECIAL EDUCATION

The U.S. Department of Education publication for parents on "Including." *(www.ed.gov/pubs/parents/Including)* "Appendix A" is an easy to understand chart of developmental milestones and the ages they're usually reached.

The Division for Early Childhood of the Council for Exceptional Children *(www.dec-sped.org).* There are links here to the various journals published by the CEC, as well as information about IDEA and special education teaching.

The Love and Learning curriculum *(www.loveandlearning.com)* was developed by parents to help their daughter, who has Down Syndrome, learn to read.

The Early Childhood Resource Center of the Research Triangle Institute *(www.rti.org/child/home.cfm)* "Supported by the latest findings in educational, psychological, behavioral, and neuroscience research, our professional consultants emphasize ways to nurture supportive relationships between very young children and the adults who care for them."

Special Education News: *(www.specialednews.com)*, a collection of news items about issues and developments in special education. You can subscribe (for free) to e-mail updates.

Exceptional Parent magazine *(www.eparent.com)* "providing information, support, ideas, encouragement and outreach for parents and families of children with disabilities and the professionals who work with them."

WOMEN'S HEALTH ISSUES

Video: Let's talk about health - What every woman should know: The GYN exam by The Arc of New Jersey (VHS videotape, 1 audiotape and 2 booklets. 1995. $28). Available from The Arc of the United States, P.O.B. 1047, Arlington, TX 76004.

Booklet: Let's talk about health - What every woman should know: The GYN exam by The Arc of New Jersey. 23 pages. 1995. (same booklet as above). 1-9 copies, $4 ea.; 10-29 copies, $3.50 ea.; over 29 copies, $3 ea. Available from The Arc of the United States, P.O.B. 1047, Arlington, TX 76004.

Research Homepage for Older Women with Disabilities *(www.uic.edu/~lisab)*

AHCPR Women's Health Highlights. Fact Sheet. AHCPR Pub. No. 98-P004, May 1998. Agency for Health Care Policy and Research, Rockville, MD. *(www.ahcpr.gov/research/womenh1.htm)*

Our Bodies, Ourselves: For The New Century. Boston Women's Health Book Collective. New York: Simon and Schuster, 1998. A book about health and sexuality written by and for women. *(www.ourbodiesourselves.org)*

Breast Health Access for Women with Disabilities *(www.salick.com/resource/features/abbreast)*

AGING

The Rehabilitation Research and Training Center on Aging with Mental Retardation. Publications and information at *www.uic.edu/orgs/rrtcamr*

Health Management of Aging Adults Who Have Mental Retardation by Ann Poindexter, MD.

RIGHTS AND RESPONSIBILITIES

HSRI, the Human Services Research Institute sponsors research and evaluation projects in the areas of deinstitutionalization, quality assurance and self-determination. You can find copies of their reports (as well as information on publications for sale) at their website *(www.hsri.org)*

Americans with Disabilities Act Document Center *(http://janweb.icdi.wvu.edu/kinder)* ADA Statute, Regulations, ADAAG (Americans with Disabilities Act Accessibility Guidelines), Federally Reviewed Tech Sheets, and Other Assistance Documents.

COMMUNITY INCLUSION

With a Little Help from My Friends, *(www.ncor.org/pcmr.htm)* an on-line booklet from the President's Committee on Mental Retardation (PCMR) has interesting chapters on a lot of the issues covered in this book.

Inclusion Daily Express *(www.inclusiondaily.com)* gives a daily digest of news items from all over the world.

The Community Imperative, a declaration supporting the right of all people with disabilities to community living *(http://soeweb.syr.edu/thechp/community_imperative.html)*. Written in 1979 by the Center on Human Policy at Syracuse University. The Center has reissued *The Community Imperative* in 2000 and invites endorsements from individuals and organizations.

Quality of Life: Perspectives and Issues, Robert L. Schalock, ed., American Association on Mental Retardation, 1990.

Interdependence: The Route to Community, Al Condeluci, GR Press, Inc., 1995.

A Brief Introduction to Social Role Valorization, Wolf Wolfensberger, Syracuse University, 1992.

ORGANIZATIONS

AAMR—American Association on Mental Retardation *(www.aamr.org)* AAMR promotes progressive policies, sound research, effective practices, and universal human rights for people with intellectual disabilities.

The ARC—*(www.thearc.org)* "The Arc of the United States is the nation's leading national organization on mental retardation. The Arc represents over seven million children and adults with mental retardation and their families. The Arc has over 140,000 members within approximately 1,000 state and local chapters nationwide."

CARF—The Rehabilitation Commission *(www.carf.org)* National accrediting body committed "To develop and maintain current, field-driven standards that improve the value and responsiveness of the programs and services delivered to people in need of rehabilitation and other life enhancement services."

The Council on Quality and Leadership in Supports for People with Disabilities *(www.thecouncil.org)* "an international organization at the forefront of the movement to create opportunities for people with disabilities. We direct our efforts toward promoting quality improvement in services and supports." Offers accreditation, quality improvement, and training based on personal outcomes.

NADD—An association for people with developmental disabilities and mental health needs *(www.thenadd.org)* NADD has been in the forefront of research and training in the area of "dual-diagnosis," treating the mental health needs of people who also have developmental disabilities.

NAMI—National Alliance of the Mentally Ill *(www.nami.org)* Politically active lobbying and information organization of families and friends of people who have mental illness. You can subscribe to an e-mail update on political issues that affect people with mental illness.

TASH *(www.tash.org)* "is an international association of people with disabilities, their family members, other advocates, and professionals fighting for a society in which inclusion of all people in all aspects of society is the norm."

ADVOCACY/SELF-ADVOCACY

The Freedom Clearinghouse *(www.freedomclearinghouse.org)*, a loose confederation of very outspoken advocacy groups. The website has links to associated groups.

Mouth *(www.mouthmag.com)* is a bi-monthly disability rights magazine whose readers' only special needs are for human rights and straight talk.

Family Village *(www.familyvillage.wisc.edu)* Sponsored by the University of Wisconsin-Madison. This is "a global community that integrates information, resources, and communication opportunities on the Internet for persons with cognitive and other disabilities, for their families, and for those that provide them services and support." This site has a Library with lots of great informational links, a Coffee Shop with links to ways people with disabilities and their families communicate with each other, and a Book Store which lists lots of relevant books, videos, audiotapes and music.

HOUSING

Opening Doors the on-line newsletter of the Technical Assistance Collaborative, Inc. *(www.tacinc.org/OpeningDoors.html)* has information about accessible and affordable housing for people with disabilities.

National Home of Your Own Alliance *(alliance.unh.edu)* , a program of the Administration of Developmental Disabilities of the US Department of Health and Human Services. Committed "to promote opportunities for people with disabilities to own and control their homes."

LIFE PLANNING

Michael Smull and ELP *(www.allenshea.com)*—articles, publications, and trainer information.

Practical Tools for Person Centered Planning, by Michael A. Mayer. Published by TheraEd *(www.theraed.com)*. Contains various assessment tools to use in discovering what people really want and need in their lives.

HISTORY

Parallels in Time, a two CD illustrated history of people with disabilities. Available from the Minnesota Governor's Council on Developmental Disabilities, 612.296.4018 or *www.comm.media.state.mn.us*

The Disability Social History Project *(www.disabilityhistory.org)*, including "Little Known Tidbits of Disability History."

A great **chronology of the disability rights movement** from Ohio State University *(www.coe.ohio-state.edu/jwheaton/rehab/chronology.htm)*

Inventing the Feeble Mind: A History of Mental Retardation in the United States, James W. Trent, Jr., University of California Press, 1994. This book is fascinating reading.

MOVIES

The following movies, available on video, give various perspectives on mental health and society.

One Flew Over the Cuckoo's Nest—Jack Nicholson as Randall Patrick McMurphy takes on The Big Nurse (or read Ken Kesey's excellent novel on which the movie was based).

The Elephant Man—based on the life of 19th Century Englishman John Merrick, this film shows how difficult it is to be accepted as a fully human being, when a disfiguring disability is the only thing people see.

Awakenings—Robin Williams awakens Robert de Niro, only to confront the limitations of drug therapy.

Being There—Peter Sellers demonstrates that "simple mindedness" may be a virtue.

What's Eating Gilbert Grape?—a young Leonardo di Caprio turns in a very convincing performance as the mentally retarded younger brother of Johnny Depp.

Rain Man—Dustin Hoffman's Raymond is a little more savvy than most people with autism, but his encounters with "the real world" make for some humorous and poignant moments.

Sling Blade—Billy Bob Thornton as an autistic man who might give community inclusion a bad name.

Star Man—This one's not really about disabilities...but the portrait of a person who has "just landed" and needs to figure out how our culture works holds many parallels with the person who has just come out of an institutional environment. Funny and sad.

The Other Sister—A little corny (isn't that the way with Hollywood), but it gives you the feeling of the enormous courage it takes for people with disabilities to insist on having their own lives in the real world.

Girl Interrupted—A good portrayal of the scary edginess that sometimes goes with mental illness and always is the result of institutionalization. "One Flew Over the Cuckoo's Nest" for girls.

I Am Sam—I cried through this whole movie. Sean Penn does a great job portraying the gut-wrenching issues of developmental disabilities and parenting.

ABOUT THE AUTHOR

James McKelvey recently retired after 25 years of support services for people with developmental disabilities. He now owns and operates "Wine & Words," a small retail shop in coastal North Carolina.

Though James holds a BA degree in Philosophy from C.W. Post College and an M.Div from Harvard, he learned support services in the late '70s as a direct care worker in a large state facility. Since then, he has worked in ICF-MR facilities, small community group homes, and specialized foster care services. In 1995 he co-founded Access, Inc., a provider of "community coaching" services in North Carolina. Access earned a 3-year accreditation from The Council on Quality and Leadership in Supports for People with Disabilities.

James' specialty has always been staff training, especially when given the opportunity to challenge old ideas and energize people to do great work. This book encapsulates years of teaching, training and support service provision. In it, James passes the torch to the next generation of people who will take support services into the 21st century.

You can contact James by e-mail: james@jamesmck.com

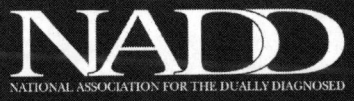

132 Fair St., Kingston, NY 12401-4802
Phone (845) 331-4336 • (800) 331-5362
Fax (845) 331-4569
e-mail: info@thenadd.org
www.thenadd.org

Join NADD today!

It's easy to sign up:
Just go to **www.thenadd.org**

Membership Matters and You Make a Difference!

Members are an integral part of what makes the National Association for the Dually Diagnosed (NADD) a leader in the dissemination of state-of-the-art information. When joining NADD you will immediately be recognized as an individual who is concerned about the issues facing mental health care for persons who have intellectual disabilities. Simply by joining NADD you will become a prestigious member and have a voice in NADD's growing influential organization.

We invite you to join NADD today and build knowledge.

NADD is the leading organization providing professionals, educators, policy makers and families with education, training and information on mental health issues relating to persons with intellectual disabilities.

Education is important and NADD provides members with opportunity to learn more:

- Regional Conferences
- Annual Conferences
- International Conferences
- Teleconference Training
- Online Training (Continuing Education Credits)
- Onsite Consulting/Training for Government/Private Organizations

NADD Members receive discounts on all services and products

Over >>

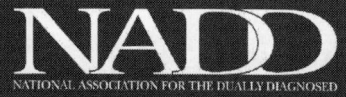

www.thenadd.org

Added Value to Your Membership

■ **Free Subscription** to *The NADD Bulletin*
Included in your membership is a subscription to *The NADD Bulletin*. Each of the six issues per year contains best practice articles by experts in the field. This publication is one of the best known resources for disseminating information on relevent issues.

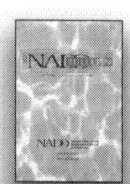

■ **Free subscription** to the *Journal of Mental Health Research in Intellectual Disabilities* (begins 2008)
The *Journal of Mental Health Rescarch in Intellectual Disabilities*, the official research journal of NADD, is soliciting articles in a variety of fields. The journal will accept a wide range of scholarly contributions with an emphasis on empirically-based research.

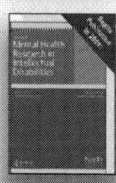

Training & Educational Products
NADD publishes the world's largest selection of training products on persons with intellectual disabilities and mental health needs including books, DVDs, CDs, videos and audiotapes.

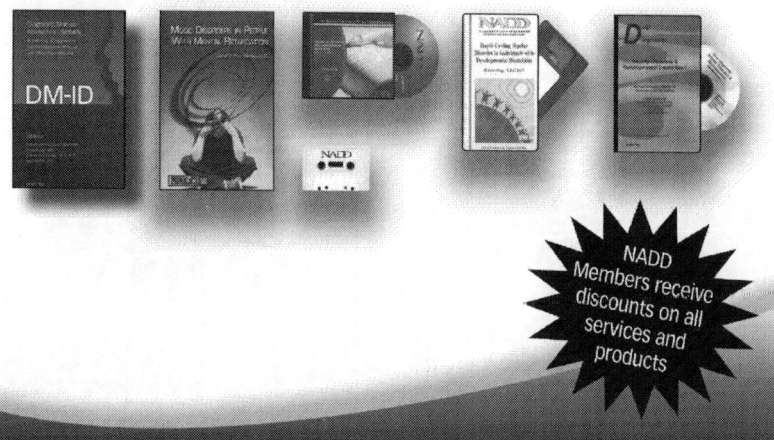

NADD Members receive discounts on all services and products